Clinical Therapy
in
Breastfeeding Patients

Clinical Therapy
in
Breastfeeding Patients

Second Edition

Thomas W. Hale, R.Ph., Ph.D.
Associate Professor of Pediatrics
Associate Professor of Pharmacology
Division of Clinical Pharmacology
Texas Tech University School of Medicine
Amarillo, Texas 79106

Pamela D. Berens, MD., FACOG
Associate Professor
Department of Obstetrics, Gynecology and Reproductive Sciences
University of Texas
Houston, Texas 77030

Clinical Therapy in Breastfeeding Patients

Second Edition

© Copyright 2002

Pharmasoft Medical Publishing

(806)-376-9900
(800)-378-1317

DISCLAIMER

ISBN 0-9636219-4-7

Preface

As the number of women who breastfeed continues to rise it is quite important that clinicians understand the various treatment protocols that are most suitable for a woman who is breastfeeding a child. Without exception, one of the most common questions we receive concerning breastfeeding mothers requiring treatment is " Which medication should we use for this mother, with this specific condition". Fortunately we have an enormous and growing source of information on drug transfer into breastmilk, but we don't always know which individual medications would be safest for the breastfeeding infant.

The purpose of this work is to provide the clinician a guide of all the various medications that may be useful for a particular medical condition, and those that are probably safest for a mother who is breastfeeding an infant. It is by no means our intent to suggest that these particular medications are *best* for the individual patient, but only that the drugs included herein have published studies on their use in breastfeeding mothers, and may be useful and safest for the particular condition in question. Many conditions require very specific medications and in some instances other drugs are simply not suitable. This is the domain of the clinician who is treating the patient and we hope a suitable medication is available and has been studied in breastfeeding mothers.

While it is quite common for clinicians to use the newest and most heavily advertised drugs, it is often these very medications that have not been studied in breastfeeding mothers. It takes time for scientists to study these medications and we suggest that often one of the older medications may be suitable for the particular condition. Fortunately many such medications are quite useful for most medical conditions.

Unfortunately, of the many thousands of medications only a small number have been fully studied in breastfeeding patients. For this reason, if a drug has no published data on its use in this population, it was excluded from this text. This does not mean that this drug cannot be used safely in breastfeeding mothers, only that we could not find any data to support its entry in this work.

Lastly, we have incorporated the new Lactation Risk Category to assist the clinician in evaluating the relative risk of the medication to the infant or breastfeeding mother.

3

Please remember that breastmilk provides an infant the most effective immunity from disease for the first year of life. The benefits of breastfeeding are enormous and now well documented so it is imperative that the infant be breastfed during the first year of life. Even brief interruptions of breastfeeding can have a significant impact on the infant and may predispose the mother to loss of milk supply. Almost invariably, a well-studied medication is available for most conditions and would be quite safe for the breastfeed dyad.

THE AUTHORS MAKE NO RECOMMENDATIONS AS TO THE SAFETY OF THESE MEDICATIONS DURING LACTATION, BUT ONLY REVIEWS WHAT IS CURRENTLY KNOWN IN THE SCIENTIFIC LITERATURE.

The references enclosed are primarily review articles that summarize the current standard of care for the various syndromes or conditions. For exact references concerning drug levels in milk please consult *Medications and Mothers' Milk* where each medication is thoroughly referenced.

Thomas W. Hale, Ph.D.
Pamela D. Berens, M.D.

How to Use this Book

Drug Name and Generic Name.
Each of the medications listed begins with their respective generic name. The Trade name refers to common trade names used in the USA.

Can/Aus/UK
Included are the most common trade names used in Canada, Australia and the United Kingdom.

Specifics
This section provides a very brief review of the drug and its levels in milk. A more thorough review is provided in the textbook, *Medications and Mothers' Milk.*

T½=
This lists the most commonly recorded adult half-life of the medication. It is very important to remember that short half-life drugs are preferred in breastfeeding mothers. Use this parameter to determine if the mother can successfully breastfeed away from the peak level of medication by nursing the infant, then taking the medication and waiting some hours for the level to drop. If the half-life is short enough (1-3 hrs), then the drug level in the maternal plasma will be declining when the infant feeds again. If the half-life is significantly long (12-24 hrs), then attempt to find a similar medication with a shorter half-life (compare ibuprofen with naproxen).

Oral=
Oral bioavailability refers to the ability of a drug to reach the systemic circulation after oral administration. It is generally a good indication of the amount of medication that is absorbed into the blood stream of the patient. Drugs with low oral bioavailability are generally either poorly absorbed in the gastrointestinal tract, or they are sequestered by the liver prior to entering the plasma compartment. The oral bioavailability listed in this text is the adult value; almost none have been published for children or neonates. Recognizing this, these values are still useful in estimating if a mother or perhaps an infant will actually absorb enough drug to provide clinically significant levels in the plasma compartment of the individual. The value listed estimates the percent of an oral dose that would be found in the plasma compartment of the individual after oral administration. In many cases, the oral bioavailability of some medications is not listed by manufacturers, but instead, terms such as "Complete", "Nil", or "Poor" are used. For lack of better data, we have included these terms when no data is available on the exact amount (percentage) absorbed.

5

Peak=
This lists the time interval from administration of the drug until it reaches the highest level in the mother's plasma, which we call the *Peak*. When the drug is at peak level in the maternal plasma it is less advisable that the mother breastfeed her infant. Rather, wait until the peak is subsiding or has at least dropped significantly before breastfeeding. Remember, drugs enter breast milk as a function of the maternal plasma concentration and the equilibrium between her plasma and milk compartments. The higher the mom's plasma level, the greater the entry of the drug into her milk. If possible, choose drugs that have short time-to-peak intervals, and suggest the mother avoid breastfeeding when the medication peaks in her plasma.

AAP:
This entry lists the recommendation provided by the American Academy of Pediatrics as published in their document, *The transfer of drugs and other chemicals into human milk (Pediatrics 108:776-789, 2001)*. Drugs are listed in tables according to the following recommendations: *Drugs that are contraindicated during breastfeeding; Drugs of abuse: Contraindicated during breastfeeding; Radioactive compounds that require temporary cessation of breastfeeding; Drugs whose effects on nursing infants is unknown but may be of concern; Drugs that have been associated with significant effects on some nursing infants and should be given to nursing mothers with caution; and Maternal medication usually compatible with breastfeeding.* In this book the AAP recommendations have been paraphrased to reflect these recommendations. "Not Reviewed" simply implies that the drug has not yet been reviewed by this committee. The author recommends that each user review these recommendations for further detail.

Lactation Risk Category (LRC):

L1   SAFEST:
Drug which has been taken by a large number of breastfeeding mothers without any observed increase in adverse effects in the infant.   Controlled studies in breastfeeding women fail to demonstrate a risk to the infant and the possibility of harm to the breastfeeding infant is remote; or the product is not orally bioavailable in an infant.

L2   SAFER:
Drug which has been studied in a limited number of breastfeeding women without an increase in adverse effects in the infant.   And/or,   the   evidence   of   a demonstrated risk   which   is   likely   to   follow   use   of   this   medication   in   a breastfeeding woman is remote.

L3 MODERATELY SAFE:
There are no controlled studies in breastfeeding women, however the risk of untoward effects to a breastfed infant is possible; or, controlled studies show only minimal non-threatening adverse effects. Drugs should be given only if the potential benefit justifies the potential risk to the infant.

L4 POSSIBLY HAZARDOUS:
There is positive evidence of risk to a breastfed infant or to breastmilk production, but the benefits from use in breastfeeding mothers may be acceptable despite the risk to the infant (e.g. if the drug is needed in a life-threatening situation or for a serious disease for which safer drugs cannot be used or are ineffective).

L5 CONTRAINDICATED:
Studies in breastfeeding mothers have demonstrated that there is significant and documented risk to the infant based on human experience, or it is a medication that has a high risk of causing significant damage to an infant. The risk of using the drug in breastfeeding women clearly outweighs any possible benefit from breastfeeding. The drug is contraindicated in women who are breastfeeding an infant.

Common Abbreviations

T½=	Adult elimination half-life
M/P	Milk/Plasma Ratio
PK=	Time to peak plasma level
Oral=	Oral bioavailability (adult)
µg/L	Microgram per liter
ng/L	Nanogram per liter
mg/L	Milligram per liter
mL	Milliliter. One cc
NSAIDs	Non-steroidal anti-inflammatory
ACEi	Angiotensin converting enzyme inhibitor
N/A	Data not available.

Table of Contents

9

Acne

Principles of Therapy:

Acne is one of the most prevalent skin diseases. It generally occurs in mid to late teens but even adults are susceptible. The etiology of the syndrome is still elusive. Acne begins in the prepubertal periods with the onset of secretion of adrenal androgens that initiate increased sebum production. Early changes in acne occur in the pilosebaceous follicles of the face and trunk with abnormal keratinization occurring in the follicular epithelium. Desquamation of the epithelial cells from follicle walls become impacted. Proliferation of anaerobic diphtheroids (*Propionibacterium acnes*) that require sebaceous lipids to grow is the next step in the inflammatory process that ensues. This bacteria subsequently releases chemo attractive factors for neutrophils that initiate the inflammatory process. Treatment of acne largely depends on the severity of symptoms but begins with therapies to suppress follicular hyperkeratosis that is the earliest event in the formation of the acne lesion. Treatments involve the use of topical agents such as tretinoin and others to suppress hyperkeratosis or antimicrobial drugs to suppress bacterial growth and subsequent inflammation. Systemic estrogens may be used in females to assist in reducing sebaceous gland secretions. While reserved for severe nodulocystic acne, isotretinoin (Accutane) is remarkably effective aside from the fact that it is horribly teratogenic (25 fold increase). Prevention of pregnancy while receiving isotretinoin and for 1 month following therapy is mandatory. Treatment of acne begins with the recognition that the disease involves not only the skin but the whole patient due largely to the many psychosocial aspects of this process

CLINDAMYCIN, TOPICAL   AAP: Compatible

Trade: Cleocin T, Clinda-Derm
Can/Aus/UK: Clindatech
Specifics: Percutaneous absorption is low (< 0.2%), breastmilk levels would be even lower. Observe for diarrhea (rare).
T½= 2.9 hours   Oral= 90%   Peak= 45-60 minutes.
LRC= L3

ERYTHROMYCIN, ORAL   AAP: Compatible

Trade: E-Mycin, Ery-Tab, Eryc, Ilosone
Can/Aus/UK: E-Mycin, Eryc, Erythromid, Novo-Rythro, PCE,Ilotyc, EMU-V, Ilosone, EES, Erythrocin, Ceplac, Erycen
Specifics: Reported milk levels are less than 1.5 mg/Liter, generally considered subclinical.
T½= 1.5-2 hours   Oral= Variable   Peak= 2-4 hours
LRC= L1

ERYTHROMYCIN+ BENZOYL PEROXIDE   **AAP:** Not Reviewed

Trade: Benzamycin
Can/Aus/UK:
Specifics: Percutaneous absorption of erythromycin or benzoyl peroxide is virtually nil.
T½= 1.5-2 hours   Oral= Variable   Peak= 2-4 hours
LRC=

ERYTHROMYCIN TOPICAL   **AAP:** Compatible

Trade: Staticin, Del-Mycin, Eryderm, T-Stat, Akne-Mycin, Erygel
Can/Aus/UK: Eryacne
Specifics: Reported milk levels following oral administration are less than 1.5 mg/Liter. They are virtually unabsorbed when administered topically.
T½= 1.5-2 hours   Oral= Variable   Peak= 2-4 hours
LRC=

TRETINOIN   **AAP:** Not Reviewed

Trade: Retin - A
Can/Aus/UK: Retin-A, Stieva-A, Vitamin A Acid, Renova, Vesanoid
Specifics: Percutaneous absorption of tretinoin is essentially nil. It is very unlikely any would enter milk.
T½= 2 hours   Oral= 70%   Peak= N/A
LRC= L3

TRIAMCINOLONE ACETONIDE   **AAP:** Not Reviewed

Trade: Tac-3, Kenalog
Can/Aus/UK: Kenalog, Triaderm, Kenacort A-10
Specifics: Intralesional injection in acne is unlikely to produce clinically relevant milk levels. Triamcinolone is considered a moderately potent steroid. It is unlikely that systemic absorption by a breastfeeding infant would be significant.
T½= 88 minutes   Oral= Complete   Peak= N/A
LRC= L3

METRONIDAZOLE TOPICAL GEL   **AAP:** Not Reviewed

Trade: MetroGel Topical
Can/Aus/UK: Metro-Gel, Metrogyl, MetroGel
Specifics: Percutaneous absorption of metronidazole is minimal.
T½= 8.5 hours   Oral= Complete   Peak= N/A
LRC= L3

ADAPALENE   AAP: Not Reviewed

Trade: Differin
Can/Aus/UK:
Specifics: Percutaneous absorption is nil. Amount in milk would be minimal.
T½= N/A   Oral= N/A   Peak= N/A
LRC= L3

AZELAIC ACID   AAP: Other

Trade: Azelex
Can/Aus/UK: Skinoren
Specifics: Percutaneous absorption is minimal (< 4%). Topical use is probably safe.
T½= N/A   Oral= N/A   Peak= N/A
LRC= L3

BENZOYL PEROXIDE   AAP: Not Reviewed

Trade: Benzac AC, Benzac W, Desquam-X, Foxtex, PanOxyl
Can/Aus/UK: Benzagel, Acetoxyl, Acnacyl, Acnecide, Acnegel
Specifics: Benzoyl peroxide activity is presumed due to release of active or free-radical oxygen capable of oxidizing bacterial proteins. It is metabolized to an inactive benzoic acid.
T½= N/A   Oral= N/A   Peak= N/A
LRC=

TAZAROTENE   AAP: Not Reviewed

Trade: Tazorac
Can/Aus/UK: Zorac
Specifics: Tazarotene is a specialized retinoid for topical use. Applied daily, it is indicated for treatment of stable plaque psoriasis of up to 20% of the body surface area. Only 2-3% of the topically applied drug is absorbed transcutaneously. Tazarotene is used for the topical treatment of stable plaque psoriasis and acne. Following topical application, tazarotene is converted to an active metabolite; transcutaneous absorption is minimal (<1%). Little compound could be detected in the plasma. However, systemic absorption is a function of the surface area. When applied to large surface areas, systemic absorption is increased. Data on transmission to breastmilk are not available.
T½=1-2 hours   Oral= N/A   Peak= 9 hours
LRC= L3

Clinical Tips:
Over emphasis on washing of the skin may actually lead to complications such as chapping and drying. Failure to cleanse the skin does not necessarily induce acne.

The topical treatment of acne with retinoids (tretinoin, tazarotene and adapalene) should be initially considered. Retinoids are poorly absorbed and milk levels are likely low if even detectable at all. Most patients can use retinoids if they begin therapy with low-strength cream formulations (0.025% tretinoin) and increase the strength later on. Other topical preparations such as the peroxides (e.g. benzoyl peroxide) are absorbed to some degree and metabolized to oxygen radicals and inactive benzoic acid byproducts almost instantly. While somewhat irritating, they are quite effective. Patients should be instructed to use cleansing agents in the morning as they have a shorter contact time and less probability of bleaching clothing. The combination of benzoyl peroxide washes in the morning and a retinoid at bedtime is a good initial therapy. Benzoyl peroxide gels and lotions should be avoided in the morning because of their bleaching of clothing during the day. The peroxides are unlikely to harm a breastfeeding infant as they are almost instantly degraded by plasma enzymes if absorbed.

Salicylic acid preparations are available but are not considered as effective as the retinoids. A new combination of benzoyl peroxide and erythromycin is popular and would not be absorbed significantly. A newer, and perhaps preferred, alternative to benzoyl peroxide is azelaic acid cream, that produces a significant reduction of *P. acnes* and an anti-keratinizing effect as well. Azelaic is only modestly absorbed via skin (< 4%), and it is rapidly metabolized. Azelaic is a normal dietary constituent in whole grains and animal products. Due to its poor penetration into plasma and rapid half-life (45 min) it is probably safe for breastfeeding mothers. Estrogens are effective therapy in reducing sebaceous gland production of lipids. If estrogens are employed in breastfeeding mothers, they should only be used a minimum of several months postpartum, in low doses, and with close observation for milk suppression. Topical antibiotic preparations include: tetracycline, metronidazole, clindamycin, erythromycin, and meclocycline sulfosalicylate. The percutaneous absorption of all the above is almost nil. In many cases plasma levels are undetectable. Therefore topical application of the above antibiotics is suitable for breastfeeding mothers. While clindamycin is commonly used, there is much resistance to erythromycin and metronidazole. However, the 'chronic' oral use of these same antibiotics is problematic. Oral tetracycline, when ingested 'in milk' is poorly bioavailable (< 30-40%). While the absolute level of tetracycline in milk is low (< 2.58 mg/Liter) and bioavailability of this would be only 30-40%, taken over a long period of time, the amount of tetracycline reaching the infant could be significant over time. The newer tetracyclines are even more problematic. The bioavailability of the newer tetracyclines (minocycline, doxycycline) is much higher (80%) even in the presence of calcium salts so that the chronic use of these tetracyclines, including minocycline and doxycycline, should be discouraged. Further, due to a chronic hypersensitivity syndrome now associated with minocycline use, most dermatologists are using doxycycline instead for chronic acne. Chronic oral therapy with clindamycin is both risky for the mother, as well as the infant, due to higher risks of pseudomembranous colitis both for the mother and infant. The use of isotretinoin (Accutane) in breastfeeding mothers is extremely risky. First, we have no data on its' use in breastfeeding mothers, but due to its high lipid solubility its transfer into milk is likely (see vitamin A). Second, the use of this incredibly teratogenic compound in a young breastfeeding mother who is at risk for pregnancy and who cannot readily use potent estrogen-containing birth control products is highly risky at best. Although controversial, some concern exists about the ability of isotretinoin to induce depression. We do not recommend the use of this product in breastfeeding mothers; the benefits of treatment do not justify the risks.

Suggested Reading:

1. Cunliffe WJ. Management of adult acne and acne variants. J Cutan Med Surg. 1998 May;2 Suppl 3:7-13. Review.
2. Webster GF. Acne and rosacea. Med Clin North Am. 1998 Sep;82(5):1145-54, vi. Review.
3. Brown SK, et al. Acne vulgaris. Lancet. 1998 Jun 20;351(9119):1871-6. Review.
4. Baur DA, et al. Current concepts in the pathogenesis and treatment of acne. J Oral Maxillofac Surg. 1998 May; 56(5):651-5. Review.
5. Usatine RP, et al. Acne vulgaris: a treatment update. Hosp Pract (Off Ed). 1998 Feb 15;33(2):111-7, 121-4, 127. Review.
6. Layton AM. Optimal management of acne to prevent scarring and psychological sequelae. Am J Clin Dermatol 2001; 2(3):135-141.
7. Jacobs DG, Deutsch NL, Brewer M. Suicide, depression, and isotretinoin: is there a causal link? J Am Acad Dermatol 2001; 45(5):S168-S175.
8. Bershad SV. The modern age of acne therapy: a review of current treatment options. Mt Sinai J Med 2001; 68(4-5) 9-286.

Allergic Rhinitis

Principles of Therapy:

Allergic rhinitis is characterized by symptoms of nasal and ocular itching, repetitive sneezing, watery rhinorrhea and nasal congestion. It is most often seasonal, occurring during spring or fall depending on the source of allergen. Perennial allergic rhinitis, which occurs independent of season, is most likely due to animal dander, house dust and insect allergens, particularly the dust mite or cockroach. Treatment of the various types of allergic rhinitis should be initially directed toward avoidance of the irritant. While significantly effective, avoidance is not always possible. Pharmacotherapy thus becomes the mainstay of treatment in most patients. Drug therapy includes the use of antihistamines, topical and oral decongestants, mast-cell stabilizers, oral or topical corticosteroids and lastly, immunotherapy. Because many of the older antihistamines are sedating (including the infant), the new non-sedating antihistamines are preferred for breastfeeding mothers. One major decongestant, phenylpropanolamine, was just removed from the US market, thus leaving only pseudoephedrine which is a problem from breast milk production. Intranasal corticosteroids may be used safely with breastfeeding mothers, as the maternal plasma levels are low, and milk levels would be virtually undetectable. Although immunotherapy has not been studied in breastfeeding mothers, the passage of minuscule levels of plant and animal proteins into milk is very unlikely.

BECLOMETHASONE   AAP: Not Reviewed

Trade: Vanceril, Beclovent, Beconase
Can/Aus/UK: Propaderm, Vanceril, Beconase, Aldecin, Becloforte, Becotide, Beclovent, Propadem
Specifics: Intrapulmonary or intranasal doses are exceedingly low and penetration into milk is extremely remote. Maternal plasma levels are virtually undetectable.
T½= 15 hours   Oral= 90%   Peak= N/A
LRC= L2

BROMPHENIRAMINE   AAP: Not Reviewed

Trade: Dimetane, Brombay, Dimetapp, Bromfed
Can/Aus/UK:
Specifics: Brompheniramine is mildly sedating. No data is available on its transfer into human milk. While not an ideal candidate, it is probably not contraindicated.
T½= 24.9 hours   Oral= Complete   Peak= 3.1 hours
LRC= L3

CETIRIZINE
AAP: Not Reviewed

Trade: Zyrtec
Can/Aus/UK: Reactine, Zyrtec
Specifics: Cetirizine is the active metabolite of hydroxyzine. Hydroxyzine has a long and safe history in infants. The fact that cetirizine is only marginally sedating is ideal.
T½= 8.3 hours   Oral= 70%   Peak= 1.7 hour
LRC= L2

CHLORPHENIRAMINE
AAP: Not Reviewed

Trade: Aller Chlor, Chlor-Tripolon, Chlor-Trimeton
Can/Aus/UK: Chlor-Tripolon, Demazin, Alunex, Piridon
Specifics: Chlorpheniramine is mildly sedating. We have no data on its transfer into human milk. While not ideal, it is probably OK to use.
T½= 12-43 hours   Oral= 25-45%   Peak= 2-6 hours
LRC= L3

CROMOLYN SODIUM
AAP: Not Reviewed

Trade: Nasalcrom, Gastrocrom, Intal
Can/Aus/UK: Nalcrom, Opticrom, Rynacrom, Vistacrom, Cromese, Intal
Specifics: Cromolyn is not systemically absorbed by the mother or the infant. It would not be orally bioavailable by the infant. It is virtually nontoxic.
T½= 80-90 minutes   Oral= < 1%   Peak= < 15 minutes
LRC= L1

FLUTICASONE
AAP: Not Reviewed

Trade: Flonase, Flovent, Cutivate
Can/Aus/UK: Flovent, Flonase, Flixotide, Flixonase
Specifics: Oral and topical absorption of fluticasone is less than 2%, so it is virtually unabsorbed. Transfer into milk is unlikely. Currently available for use in infants.
T½= 7.8 hours   Oral= Inhaled(30%)   Peak= 15-60 minutes
LRC= L3

MOMETASONE
AAP: Not Reviewed

Trade: Nasonex
Can/Aus/UK:
Specifics: It is extremely unlikely mometasone would be excreted into

17

human milk in clinically relevant levels following topical or intranasal administration.

T½= N/A   Oral= N/A   Peak= N/A
LRC= L3

LORATADINE   AAP: Not Reviewed

Trade: Claritin
Can/Aus/UK: Claritin, Claratyne, Clarityn
Specifics: Only minimal amounts are transferred into human milk.
T½= 8.4-28 hours   Oral= Complete   Peak= 1.5 hours
LRC= L2

PHENYLPROPANOLAMINE   AAP: Not Reviewed

Trade: Dexatrim, Acutrim
Can/Aus/UK:
Specifics: While the transfer of phenylpropanolamine into human milk is unknown, it is a common ingredient in pediatric cold formulas although it has been removed from the market in the USA.   The amount available in milk is probably subclinical.
T½= 5.6 hours   Oral= 100%   Peak= 1 hour
LRC= L2

PSEUDOEPHEDRINE   AAP: Compatible

Trade: Sudafed, Halofed, Novafed, Actifed
Can/Aus/UK: Eltor, Pseudofrin, Sudafed, Balminil, Contac
Specifics: Absolute levels of pseudoephedrine in milk are very low. However, new unpublished data from our laboratories suggests that pseudoephedrine may suppress milk production significantly(approx. 21%). Long term use may suppress milk output and should be avoided.
T½= < 4 hours   Oral= 90%   Peak= 0.5-1 hours
LRC= L3 for acute use
          L4 for chronic use

TRIPROLIDINE   AAP: Compatible

Trade: Actidil
Can/Aus/UK:
Specifics: Triprolidine is mildly sedating. Milk levels are extremely low.
T½= 5 hours   Oral= Complete   Peak= 2 hours
LRC= L1

PHENYLEPHRINE   AAP: Not Reviewed

Trade: Neo-synephrine, AK-dilate
Can/Aus/UK:
Specifics: There are no data on the transfer of phenylephrine into milk, however, poor oral bioavailability would limit dose to infant. No untoward effects have yet been reported via milk.
T½= 2-3 hours   Oral= 38%   Peak= 10-60 minutes
LRC= L3

AZELASTINE   AAP: Not Reviewed

Trade: Astelin
Can/Aus/UK:
Specifics: There are no data on the transfer of azelastine into milk, however, poor intranasal bioavailability would limit dose to infant when used in this dosage form. No untoward effects have yet been reported via milk.
T½= 22-25 hours   Oral= 40% intranasal   Peak= 10-60 minutes
LRC=

OXYMETAZOLINE   AAP: Not Reviewed

Trade: Afrin nasal spray
Can/Aus/UK:
Specifics: There are no data on the transfer of oxymetazoline into milk, however, significant intranasal absorption has been reported with systemic side effects in users. Occasional short-term use is probably OK, but avoid chronic use absolutely. Nasal absorption is negligible.
T½= 5-8 hours   Oral= N/A   Peak= 10-60 minutes
LRC=

Clinical Tips:

While antihistamines have been used in infants and breastfeeding mothers for many years, the clinician should attempt to use the newer non-sedating varieties as sedation in breastfed infants may increase the risk of SIDS. Astemizole has a long half-life, numerous drug-drug interactions and has been reported to induce sedation in breastfed infants and should be avoided. Clemastine has been reported to induce drowsiness, irritability, refusal to feed and neck stiffness and should be avoided. Chlorpheniramine and brompheniramine are probably safe to use but should be avoided for long-term therapy due to sedation of the infant. While diphenhydramine(Benadryl) has been used for many years both in infants and breastfeeding mothers, its ability to induce sedation makes it less ideal for long-term therapy in breastfed infants. Its short-term use is safe in normal (non-apneic) infants. Current data suggest loratadine and cetirizine are preferred antihistamines due to minimal sedation and their documented safe use in infants. A newer non-sedating antihistamine azelastine (Astelin) may be useful when used intra nasally, as it poorly absorbed (only 40%) and has minimal side effects. However, we do not have breastfeeding data as of yet on this product. Oral decongestants including phenylephrine, and phenylpropanolamine, have been used for many years in breastfeeding mothers, largely without reported side effect although phenylpropranolamine was recently removed from the US market due to cardiovascular toxicity. Recent data from our laboratories suggests that pseudoephedrine may significantly suppress milk production in some mothers, particularly those long postpartum. While it may be useful for engorgement and for short-term use, long-term use may suppress milk production and lead to reduced weight gain in infants. While the other decongestants transfer into milk to some degree, they have not been reported to produce significant problems. Nevertheless, they should only be used on a short term basis. Topical, intranasal decongestant sprays such as oxymetazoline and naphazoline have not been studied in breastfeeding mothers but their plasma levels while not high at recommended doses can lead to adrenergic side effects if overdosed. While the intranasal absorption is reported as significant, no oral data seems to be available so the oral absorption in a breastfeeding infant may or may not be possible. Regardless, it is not overly likely that the amount of oxymetazoline or naphazoline absorbed via the nasal mucosa would cause overt side effects in a breastfed infant. But rebound congestion and a syndrome called *rhinitis medicamentosa*, in which a progressively shorter duration of action leads to continuous use, is well known and patients are generally advised to avoid chronic use of these medications. Cromolyn is virtually nontoxic and non-absorbed. It is unlikely to produce untoward effects in a breastfed infant. At present we do not have data on the topical use of nasal steroids in breastfeeding women. Of the group fluticasone is not bioavailable and therefore would be an ideal choice. Further, it cleared for use in young infants. Although we do not have data on the other nasal steroids(triamcinolone,mometasone, budesonide, beclomethasone), most are unlikely to transfer to human milk in clinically relevant amounts if normal therapeutic doses are used by the mother. Of the above remedies, maternal use of cromolyn and the topical nasal steroids are the least likely to produce long-term problems in breastfed infants.

Suggested Reading:

1.   Nash DR. Allergic rhinitis. Pediatr Ann. 1998 Dec;27(12):799-808. Review.
2.   Meltzer EO. Pharmacological treatment options for allergic rhinitis and asthma. Clin Exp Allergy. 1998 Jun;28 Suppl 2:27-36. Review.
3.   Urval KR. Overview of diagnosis and management of allergic rhinitis. Prim Care. 1998 Sep;25(3):649-62. Review.
4.   Allergic rhinitis. Harv Womens Health Watch. 1998 May;5(9):2-3. Review.
5.   Cook PR. Allergic rhinitis. Outcomes of immunotherapy on symptom control. Otolaryngol Clin North Am. 1998 Feb;31(1):129-40. Review.
6.   Tripathi A, Patterson R. Impact of allergic rhinitis treatment on quality of life. Pharmacoeconomics 2001; 19(9):891-899.

7. Nielsen LP, Mygind N, Dahl R. Intranasal corticosteroids for allergic rhinitis: superior relief? Drugs 2001; 61(11):1563-1579.
8. Berger WE. Treatment update: allergic rhinitis. Allergy Asthma Proc 2001; 22(4):191-198.

Anesthetic Agents

Principles of Therapy:

Medications used in anesthesia comprise an unusual array of compounds, consisting of those with local effects such as lidocaine or bupivacaine, those with widespread systemic effects such as the benzodiazepines, opioid analgesics and gaseous general anesthetics. Although the data concerning many of these products and their transfer into human milk is still rather limited, there are data on most of these medications. It is important to remember that virtually all medications transfer into human milk to some degree. The absolute amount of transfer of drugs into milk is determined largely by equilibrium forces between the maternal plasma and the milk compartment. Because many anesthetic medications have brief plasma half-lives and rapidly redistribute from the plasma compartment to other remote compartments(adipose, muscle), the overall degree of exposure of the breastfeeding infant via breastmilk is often quite minimal. Because of this rapid redistribution from the plasma to other compartments in breastfeeding mothers, most anesthetic drugs attain minimal levels in milk. The anesthetic agents that follow have been studied in breastfeeding mothers and their milk levels are for the most part quite low. As such, they are unlikely to induce clinical effects in a breastfeeding infant.

ALFENTANIL   AAP: Not Reviewed

    Trade: Alfenta
    Can/Aus/UK: Alfenta, Rapifen
    Specifics: Following a dose of 50 µg/kg IV, the mean levels of alfentanil in colostrum at 4 hours varied from 0.21 to 1.56 µg/L of milk, levels probably too small to produce overt toxicity in breastfeeding infants. In another study following a dose of 50 micrograms or more, breastmilk levels were 0.88 µg/Liter at 4 hours and 0.05 µg/Liter at 28 hours.
    T½= 1-2 hours   Oral= N/A   Peak= Immediate
    LRC= L2

BUPIVACAINE   AAP: Compatible

    Trade: Marcaine
    Can/Aus/UK: Marcaine
    Specifics: In one study of five patients, levels of bupivacaine in breastmilk were below the limits of detection (< 0.02 mg/L) at 2 to 48 hours postpartum. These authors concluded that bupivacaine is a safe drug for perinatal use in mothers who plan to breastfeed.
    T½= 2.7 hours   Oral= N/A   Peak= 30-45 minutes
    LRC= L2

DIAZEPAM   **AAP:** May be of concern

Trade: Valium
Can/Aus/UK: Apo-Diazepam, Meval, Novo-Dipam, Vivol, Antenex, Ducene, Valium, Sedapam
Specifics: In a study of 9 mothers receiving diazepam postpartum, milk levels of diazepam varied from approximately 0.01 to 0.08 mg/L. Taken together, most studies suggest that the dose of diazepam and its metabolite, desmethyldiazepam, to a suckling infant will be on average 5% and at a maximum 12% of the weight-adjusted maternal dose of diazepam. While chronic use could lead to buildup in an infant, the acute use of one or two doses is unlikely to produce sedation in an infant.
T½= 43 hours   Oral= Complete   Peak= 1-2 hours
LRC= L3
     L4 if used chronically

FENTANYL   **AAP:** Compatible

Trade: Sublimaze
Can/Aus/UK: Sublimaze, Duragesic
Specifics: The transfer of fentanyl into human milk is extremely low. In a group of ten women receiving a total dose of 50 to 400 µg fentanyl IV during labor, the concentration of fentanyl in milk was exceedingly low, generally below the level of detection (<0.05 ng/mL).
T½= 2-4 hours   Oral= 25-75%   Peak=7-8 minutes (IV)
LRC= L2

GLYCOPYRROLATE   **AAP:** Not Reviewed

Trade: Robinul
Can/Aus/UK: Robinul
Specifics: After administration, its plasma half-life is exceedingly short (< 5 minutes) with most of the product being distribution out of the plasma compartment rapidly. No data on transfer into human milk is available, but due to its short plasma half-life, and its quaternary structure, it is very unlikely that significant quantities would penetrate milk.
T½= 1.7 hours   Oral= 10-25%   Peak= 5 hours (oral)
LRC= L3

HALOTHANE   **AAP:** Compatible

Trade: Fluothane
Can/Aus/UK: Fluothane
Specifics: Approximately 60-80% is rapidly eliminated by exhalation the first 24 hours postoperative, and only 15% is actually metabolized by the liver.

After a 3 hour surgery, only 2 ppm was detected in milk. At another exposure in one week, only 0.83 and 1.9 ppm were found. The authors assessed the exposure to the infant as negligible.

T½= N/A   Oral= N/A   Peak= 10-20 minutes
LRC= L2

KETOROLAC   AAP: Compatible

Trade: Toradol, Acular
Can/Aus/UK: Acular, Toradol
Specifics: In a study of 10 patients receiving 10 mg PO four times daily ketorolac was undetectable in 4 milk samples, and exceedingly low in the other 6 patient samples (5.2-7.3 µg/L). While the manufacturer does not approve use in breastfeeding mothers, the levels in breastmilk are incredibly low, far too low to induce clinical effects in a breastfeeding infant. No evidence of untoward effects in infants has been published.

T½= 2.4-8.6 hours   Oral= >81%   Peak= 0.5 - 1 hr.
LRC= L2

LIDOCAINE   AAP: Compatible

Trade: Xylocaine
Can/Aus/UK: Xylocard, Xylocaine, Lignocaine, EMLA
Specifics: In one study of a breastfeeding mother who received IV lidocaine for ventricular arrhythmias, the mother received approximately 965 mg over 7 hours including the bolus starting doses. At seven hours, breastmilk samples were drawn and the concentration of lidocaine was 0.8 mg/L, or 40% of the maternal plasma level (2.0 mg/L). Assuming that the mother's plasma was maintained at 5µg/mL (therapeutic = 1.5-5µg/mL), an infant consuming 1 L per day of milk would ingest approximately 2 mg/day, which would be subclinical.

T½= 1.8 hours   Oral= < 35%   Peak= Immediate(IV)
LRC= L3

LORAZEPAM   AAP: Compatible

Trade: Ativan
Can/Aus/UK: Apo-Lorazepam, Ativan, Novo-Lorazepam, Almazine
Specifics: In one patient receiving 2.5 mg twice daily for 5 days postpartum, the breastmilk levels were 12 µg/L. In another patient four hours after an oral dose of 3.5 mg, milk levels averaged 8.5 µg/L. It would appear from these studies that the amount of lorazepam secreted into milk would be clinically insignificant under most conditions..

T½= 2.2 hours   Oral= 60-75%   Peak= 1 hour
LRC= L3

MEPERIDINE / PETHIDINE

AAP: Not Reviewed

Trade: Demerol
Can/Aus/UK: Demerol, Pethidine,
Specifics: In a study of 9 nursing mothers two hours after a 50 mg IM injection, the concentration of meperidine in breastmilk was 0.13 mg/L. In another study of two nursing mothers, the concentration of meperidine 8-12 hours following a dose of 150 or 75 mg was 0.209 and 0.275 mg/L respectively. Long-term use may produce higher levels of the metabolite normeperidine, which has a long half-life (63-73 hours).
T½= 3.2 hours   Oral= <50%   Peak= 30-50 min (IM)
LRC= L2
          L3 if used early postpartum

METOCLOPRAMIDE

AAP: Compatible

Trade: Reglan
Can/Aus/UK: Apo-Metoclop, Emex, Maxeran, Reglan, Maxolon, Pramin, Gastromax, Paramid
Specifics: Peak metoclopramide levels in milk occur at 2-3 hours after administration of the medication. During the late puerperium, the concentration of metoclopramide in the milk varied from 20 to 125µg/L, which was less than the 28 to 157µg/L noted during the early puerperium. The authors estimated the daily dose to infant to vary from 6 to 24µg/kg/day during the early puerperium, and from 1 to 13µg/kg/day during the late phase. These doses are minimal compared to those used for therapy of reflux in pediatric patients (0.1 to 0.5 mg/kg/day). In these studies, only 1 of 5 infants studied had detectable blood levels of metoclopramide, hence no accumulation or side effects were observed.
T½= 5-6 hours   Oral= 30-100%   Peak= 1-2 hours
LRC= L2

MIDAZOLAM

AAP: May be of concern

Trade: Versed
Can/Aus/UK: Versed, Hypnovel
Specifics: After oral administration of 15 mg for up to 6 days postnatally in 22 women, the mean milk/plasma ratio was 0.15 and the maximum level of midazolam in breastmilk was 9 nanogram/mL and occurred 1-2 hours after administration. After IV use, it is rapidly distributed out of the plasma compartment. Milk levels would be minimal.
T½= 2-5 hours   Oral= 60-75%   Peak= 20-50 min
LRC= L3

MORPHINE   AAP: Compatible

Trade: Morphine
Can/Aus/UK: Epimorph,   Morphitec,   M.O.S.,   MS   Contin,   Statex,
Morphalgin, Ordine, Anamorph, Kapanol, Oramorph, Sevredol
Specifics: In a group of 5 lactating women,   the highest morphine
concentration in breastmilk following two epidural doses was only 82µg/L at
30 minutes. The highest breastmilk level following 15 mg IV/IM was only 0.5
mg/L. In another study of women receiving morphine via PCA pumps for 12-
48 hours postpartum, the concentration of morphine in breastmilk ranged
from 50-60µg/L..
T½= 1.5-2 hours   Oral= 26%   Peak= 0.5-1 hr.
LRC= L3

NALBUPHINE   AAP: Not Reviewed

Trade: Nubain
Can/Aus/UK: Nubain
Specifics: In a group of 20 postpartum mothers who received 20 mg IM
nalbuphine,   the total amount of nalbuphine excreted into human milk during
a 24 hour period averaged 2.3 micrograms, which is equivalent to 0.012% of
the maternal dosage. The mean milk/plasma ratio using the AUC was 1.2.
According to the authors, an oral intake of 2.3 micrograms nalbuphine would
not produce any measurable plasma concentrations in the neonate.
T½= 5 hours   Oral= 16%   Peak=2-15min (IV,IM)
LRC= L3

NITROUS OXIDE   AAP: Not Reviewed

Trade:
Can/Aus/UK: Entonox
Specifics: Nitrous oxide has a plasma half-life of < 3 minutes and is rapidly
eliminated from the body. It would not likely enter milk nor be orally
bioavailable to an infant.
T½= < 3 minutes   Oral= Nil   Peak= N/A
LRC= L3

PROPOFOL   AAP: Not Reviewed

Trade: Diprivan
Can/Aus/UK: Diprivan
Specifics: In one study of 3 women who received propofol 2.5 mg/kg IV
followed by a continuous infusion, the breastmilk levels ranged from 0.04 to
0.74 mg/L.   The second breastmilk level obtained 24 hours after delivery
contained only 6% of the 4-hour sample. Similar levels (0.12-0.97 mg/L)

were noted in colostrum samples obtained 4-8 hours after induction with propofol. From these data it is apparent that only minimal levels of propofol is transferred to human milk.

T½= 1-3 days   Oral= N/A   Peak=immediate (IV)
LRC= L2

THIOPENTAL SODIUM   **AAP:** Compatible

Trade: Pentothal
Can/Aus/UK: Pentothal, Intraval
Specifics: Thiopental is an ultra-short acting barbiturate sedative and rapidly distributes to muscle and adipose tissue. Thiopental sodium is secreted into milk in low levels. In a study of two groups of 8 women who received from 5.0 to 5.4 mg/Kg thiopental sodium, the maximum concentration in breastmilk 0.9 mg/L in mature milk and in colostrum was 0.34 mg/L. The milk/plasma ratio was 0.3 for colostrum and 0.4 for mature milk. The maximum daily dose to infant would be 0.135 mg/kg or approximately 3% of the adult dose.

T½= 3-8 hours (elimination) Oral= variable   Peak= immediate
LRC= L3

Clinical Tips:

Because most anesthetic agents are used for only brief periods, the absolute dose transferred into breastmilk is usually extremely low. Drugs are, without exception, transferred from the plasma compartment of the mother directly into the breast milk. In general, agents that do not attain high levels in the plasma compartment do not attain high levels in the milk compartment. In addition, medications that are rapidly redistributed from the plasma to peripheral compartments do not usually produce high concentrations in milk either. Many anesthetic agents are rapidly cleared from the maternal plasma within minutes because they are redistributed to deep tissue compartments. Therefore both the duration and degree of breastmilk exposure is very brief. For this reason, the absolute daily dose transferred into milk is almost always low. This is fortuitous for breastfeeding mothers, as most all the literature thus far clearly suggests that the absolute amount of anesthetic agents transferred into human milk is below clinical relevance. Based on the present literature, the early return to breastfeeding is advisable and advantageous for both mother and infant.

All of the above anesthetic agents have been studied in breastfeeding mothers. Most of these medications are only used once during the procedure, thus the volume of distribution is not filled at all. Because of this rapid redistribution, plasma levels of many of these agents are low and fleeting. For this reason, most all of the current studies indicate that milk levels are very low or barely detectable. Thus far, with exception of morphine, meperidine and diazepam, we do not have any data suggesting that these agents transfer into milk in clinically relevant amounts. Many anesthesiologists now recommend that as soon as a mother feels awake and alert, she can breastfeed. It is important to remember that the transport of drugs into milk is difficult, and most drugs penetrate milk poorly. However, it is always important to consider the age and stability of the infant. In a premature or weakened infant, the clinician may opt to hold breastfeeding for a few hours to reduce the risk in certain circumstances. In a healthy fullterm, or older infant, these medications are not likely to produce any major side effects. General recommendations for anesthesia in breastfeeding mothers are:

Premedication. Therapeutic doses of temazepam, lorazepam, midazolam, opioids and glycopyrrolate may be safely used. Preferred H_2 blockers include ranitidine or famotidine.

Induction. Thiopental sodium, or propofol have both been shown to be safe.

Muscle Relaxants. We have little data on these agents, but thus far no untoward effects have been reported.

Antinauseants: We do not yet have breastmilk levels on ondansetron or granisetron although they are routinely used in pediatric oncology. It is unlikely their milk levels will be high enough to induce clinical effects in a breastfeeding infant. Metoclopramide has been extensively studied and is largely without clinical effect in a breastfed infant.

Postoperative analgesia. Preferred opiates vary with the procedure but morphine, fentanyl, sufentanil or others may be used safely. Meperidine has been implicated in neonatal sedation and behavioral delay and should be used cautiously. NSAIDs of choice include ketorolac, ibuprofen, or diclofenac. Kappa opioids such as nalbuphine(Nubain) can be used safely in postpartum women, as milk levels are low. In infants with respiratory difficulties, opioids should be use cautiously.

Local anesthetics. Thus far without exception, the transfer of local anesthetics into human milk has been extremely low in those studied. Studies with lidocaine[6,7] and bupivacaine show milk levels to be subclinical. While ropivacaine is gaining in popularity due to its reduced hypotensive, cardiotoxic and CNS side effects in patients we still do not have data on its transfer to human milk.

Suggested Reading:

1. Wittels BK, Scott DT, Sinatra RS: Exogenous opioids in human breast milk and acute neonatal neuro behavior: a preliminary study. Anesthesiology 1990; 73:864-869.
2. Spigset O: Anaesthetic agents and excretion in breast milk. Acta Anaesthesiologica Scandinavica 1994; 38:94-103.
3. Lee JJ. And Rubin A.P. Breast feeding and anesthesia. Anaesthesia 48:616-625, 1993.
4. Giuliani M, Grossi GB, Pileri M, Lajolo C, Casparrini G. Could local anesthesia while breast-feeding be harmful to infants? J Pediatr Gastroenterol Nutr 2001; 32(2):142-144.

5. Ransjo-Arvidson AB, Matthiesen AS, Lilja G, Nissen E, Widstrom AM, Uvnas Moberg K. Maternal analgesia during labor disturbs newborn behavior: effects on breastfeeding, temperature, and crying. Birth 2001; 28(1):5-12.

6. Schneider P, Reinhold P. [Anesthesia in breast feeding. Which restrictions are justified?] Anasthesie in der Stillzeit. Welche Einschrankungen sind gerechtfertigt? Anasthesiol Intensivmed Notfallmed Schmerzther 2000; 35(6):356-374.

7. Dryden RM, Lo MW. Breast milk lidocaine levels in tumescent liposuction. Plast Reconstr Surg 2000; 105(6):2267-2268.

8. Hale TW. Anesthetic medications in breastfeeding mothers. J Hum Lact 1999; 15(3):185-194.

9. Hirose M, Hara Y, Hosokawa T, Tanaka Y. The effect of postoperative analgesia with continuous epidural bupivacaine after cesarean section on the amount of breast feeding and infant weight gain. Anesth Analg 1996; 82(6):1166-1169.

Angina Pectoris

Principles of Therapy:

Angina pectoris is precordial chest pain, usually associated with exercise and is rapidly relieved by rest or nitrates. The typical definition of angina pectoris is that of transient discomfort in the chest, arm, jaw, back or shoulder which is provoked by exercise or excitement and is relieved by nitrates.   Angina is usually due to myocardial ischemia secondary to poor vascular supply in the myocardium. Regardless of the etiology, myocardial ischemia occurs when there is an imbalance between oxygen supply via the coronary arteries, and myocardial oxygen demand. In stable angina patients, the major etiology of the angina is probably increased oxygen demand.   However, in unstable angina, a decreased myocardial oxygen supply results from interruptions of blood supply such as following thrombus formation, platelet aggregation and/or vasoconstriction.   Classic methods of treatment of angina include reducing the heart rate, blood pressure, peripheral resistance, workload on the heart and vascular spasms. Ultimately, most of the medications used reduce the workload on the heart with only minimal changes in overall oxygen supply to the myocardium.

METOPROLOL   **AAP:** Compatible

Trade: Toprol XL, Lopressor
Can/Aus/UK: Apo-Metoprolol, Betaloc, Lopressor, Novo-Metoprol, Minax,
Specifics: First line choice of beta-blocker for breastfeeding women. Milk levels are minimal. Side effects in infant are minimal.
T½= 3-7 hours   Oral= 40-50%   Peak= 2.5-3 hours
LRC= L3

NIFEDIPINE   **AAP:** Compatible

Trade: Adalat, Procardia
Can/Aus/UK: Adalat, Apo-Nifed, Novo-Nifedin, Nu-Nifed, Nifecard, Nyefax, Nefensar XL
Specifics: Milk levels of this calcium channel blocker are quite low. Its use in angina is not preferred.
T½= 1.8-7 hours   Oral= 50%   Peak= 45 min-4 hours
LRC= L2

PROPRANOLOL   **AAP:** Compatible

Trade: Inderal
Can/Aus/UK: Detensol, Inderal, Novo-Pranol, Deralin, Cardinol
Specifics: Propranolol is an ideal beta-blocker for breastfeeding women.

Numerous studies show minimal milk levels and minimal to no side effects in the infant.

T½= 3-5 hours   Oral= 30%   Peak= 60-90 min.
LRC= L3

VERAPAMIL   **AAP:** Compatible

Trade: Calan, Isoptin, Covera-HS
Can/Aus/UK: Apo-Verap, Isoptin, Novo-Veramil, Anpec, Veracaps SR, Berkatens, Cordilox, Univer
Specifics: Verapamil levels in milk are generally quite low, and side effects have not been noted in breastfeeding infants. Verapamil may also be used in panic and manic attacks. But because it reduces uterine contractility, discontinue prior to delivery.

T½= 3-7 hours   Oral= 90%   Peak= 1-2.2
LRC= L2

NITROGLYCERINE   **AAP:** Not Reviewed

Trade: Nitrong, Nitro-Bid, Nitroglyn
Can/Aus/UK: Nitrong SR, Nitrol, Transderm-Nitro, Nitro-Dur, Anginine, Nitrolingual Spray, Nitradisc, Deponit
Specifics: No data are available on the transfer of nitroglycerin into milk, but some caution is urged. Oral nitroglycerine bioavailability is < 1%, sublingually 38%, and topically 72%. So the method of administration is important to the overall bioavailability of the product.

T½= 1-4 minutes   Oral= Variable   Peak= 2-20 minutes
LRC= L4

DALTEPARIN SODIUM   **AAP:** Not Reviewed

Trade: Fragmin, Low Molecular Weight Heparin
Can/Aus/UK:
Specifics: In another study of 15 post-caesarian patients following subcutaneous doses of 2500 IU, maternal plasma levels averaged 0.074 to 0.308 IU/mL. Breastmilk levels of dalteparin ranged from < 0.005 to 0.037 IU/mL of milk. Using this data, an infant ingesting 150 mL/kg/day would ingest approximately 5.5 IU/kg/day. Due to the polysaccharide nature of this production, oral absorption is unlikely. The authors suggested that "It appears highly unlikely that puerperal thromboprophylaxis with LMWH has any clinically relevant effect on the nursing infant."

T½= 2.3 hours   Oral= None   Peak= 2-4 hours (SC)
LRC= L2

ENOXAPARIN   **AAP:** Not Reviewed

Trade: Lovenox, Low Molecular Weight Heparin
Can/Aus/UK: Clexane, Lovenox
Specifics: Enoxaparin is a low molecular-weight fraction of heparin used clinically as an anticoagulant. In a study of 12 women receiving 20-40 mg of enoxaparin daily for up to 5 days postpartum for venous pathology (n=4) or caesarian section (n=8), no change in anti-Xa activity was noted in the breastfed infants. Because it is a peptide fragment of heparin, its molecular weight is large (2000-8000 daltons). The size alone would largely preclude its entry into human milk at levels clinically relevant. Due to minimal oral bioavailability, any present in milk would not be orally absorbed by the infant.

T½= 4.5 hours   Oral= None   Peak= 3-5 hours (SC)
LRC= L3

TINZAPARIN   **AAP:** Not Reviewed

Trade: Innohep
Can/Aus/UK: Innohep
Specifics: Tinzaparin is a low molecular weight heparin with antithrombotic properties used for the treatment of deep vein thrombosis. No data are available on its transfer to milk. However, due to its protein nature and its large molecular weight, breastmilk levels would be expected to be quite low. Some breastfeeding data are available for a similar product, dalteparin.

T½= 2.3 hours   Oral= None   Peak= 2-4 hours (SC)
LRC= L3

ASPIRIN   **AAP:** May be of concern

Trade: Aspirin, Ecotrin, Excedrin
Can/Aus/UK: Ecotrin
Specifics: Aspirin levels in human milk are exceedingly low. Occasional use in breastfeeding mothers is not absolutely contraindicated. It should never be used when the infant is sick or febrile, due to its relationship with Reye's syndrome.

T½= 2.5-7 hours   Oral= 80-100%   Peak= 1-2 hours
LRC= L3

Clinical Tips:

The primary goal of treatment is to reduce either the workload on the heart or reduce the etiology of reduced blood supply such as infarct. Although eliminating anginal symptoms is a stated goal, simply abolishing angina may not be effective in prolonging patient survival. The major goal must therefore be to eliminate the reason for myocardial ischemia. In essence, pharmacotherapy generally consists of multiple avenues of attack and includes beta-blockers, nitrates and calcium channel blockers. The beta-blockers have for years been important in reducing myocardial ischemia as they generally reduce total peripheral resistance, thus reducing overall workload on the heart. The goal of beta-blocker therapy is to lower the resting heart rate to 50-60 beats/minute. Atenolol, propranolol, metoprolol, labetalol and carvedilol all seem to be effective in reducing myocardial ischemia. Pindolol has been documented to be ineffective and should not be used in ischemic patients. Of these agents, most have been studied in breastfeeding patients.

Propranolol reduces anginal pain by reducing heart rate and probably blood pressure. Propranolol is transferred into milk in extremely low amounts and is an ideal beta-blocker for breastfeeding mothers. Metoprolol levels in breastmilk are also quite low and it is more cardioselective. While some side effects in breastfed infants have been noted with atenolol, it is probably safe when used judiciously. Observe infants for sedation, apnea, and hypoglycemia if long-term, higher doses are used. Of the beta-blockers, avoid acebutolol and perhaps atenolol. Of the calcium channel blockers, nifedipine is the least preferred due to questioned efficacy although it transfers into milk minimally. Numerous other calcium channel blockers are available but most have not been studied in this syndrome. Diltiazem has been found effective, but its transfer into milk is significant and caution is recommended. At present, we have no data on the transfer of nitroglycerin into human milk, but nitrates present in water have been found to transfer into milk poorly and are not contraindicated. While some caution is recommended with nitrates, until we get more data, they are not likely to cause overt side effects in infants. Due to the extremely short half-life of nitroglycerin, a brief interval prior to breastfeeding(2-3 hours) would probably eliminate any risk. Long-acting nitrates (isosorbide dinitrate) are subject to tolerance and may not justify the risk to the breastfeeding infant.

Antiplatelet agents such as ticlopidine and clopidogrel have been poorly studied and are not necessarily more effective than aspirin. Long-term aspirin therapy in breastfeeding mothers is generally not recommended. Data from the last decade clearly suggest that aspirin may significantly increase the risk of Reye's syndrome in infants. Although milk levels of aspirin are extraordinarily low, it should probably not be used in breastfeeding mothers for long periods. Low molecular weight heparins such as enoxaparin, tinzaparin and dalteparin are presently popular and have been found to significantly reduce MI, recurrent angina, and death in patients with unstable angina. New data also suggests that dalteparin levels in milk (5.5 IU/Kg/day) are extraordinarily low and would not affect a nursing infant. This is not unexpected, as they are large molecular weight proteins and would not be bioavailable even if ingested by the infant.

Suggested Reading:

1.   Asirvatham S, et al. Choosing the most appropriate treatment for stable angina. Safety considerations. Drug Saf. 1998 Jul;19(1):23-44. Review.

2. Parmley WW. Optimum treatment of stable angina pectoris. Cardiovasc Drugs Ther. 1998 Apr;12 Suppl 1:105-10. Review.

3. McKenna CJ, et al. Current management of chronic stable angina. Ir Med J. 1998 May-Jun;91(3):85. Review.

4. Staniforth AD. Evidence based treatment of chronic stable angina. Int J Cardiol. 1998 Jan 5;63(1):21-5. Review.

5. Parker JD, et al. Nitrate therapy for stable angina pectoris. N Engl J Med. 1998 Feb 19;338(8):520-31. Review.

6. Wlodek L, Sokolowska M. [Why does nitroglycerin tolerance appear?] Dlaczego pojawia sie tolerancja na nitrogliceryne? Postepy Hig Med Dosw 2001; 55(5):673-685.

7. Collet JP, Choussat R, Montalescot G. [Review and future perspectives on low-molecular-weight heparin] Acquis et perspectives des heparines de bas poids moleculaire. Arch Mal Coeur Vaiss 2001; 94(11 Suppl):1233-1242.

8. Aronow WS. Drug treatment of elderly patients with acute myocardial infarction: practical recommendations. Drugs Aging 2001; 18(11):807-818.

9. Davies SW. Clinical presentation and diagnosis of coronary artery disease: stable angina. Br Med Bull 2001; 59:17-27.

10. Blackwell M, Huckell V, Turek MA. The medical management of acute coronary syndromes and chronic ischemic heart disease in women. Can J Cardiol 2001; 17 Suppl D:49D-52D.

11. Sica DA. Current concepts of pharmacotherapy in hypertension: combination calcium channel blocker therapy in the treatment of hypertension. J Clin Hypertens (Greenwich) 2001; 3(5):322-327.

12. Schulman SP, Fessler HE. Management of acute coronary syndromes. Am J Respir Crit Care Med 2001; 164(6):917-922.

Anticoagulation Therapy

Principles of Therapy:

Long-term anticoagulation therapy is becoming increasingly common for a widening range of illnesses. Due to the efficacy of anticoagulant therapy in ischemic syndromes as well as in syndromes with atrial fibrillation and arrhythmias, the number of patients undergoing chronic anticoagulant therapy has risen. The number of agents used to inhibit coagulation has increased as well, with introduction of the newer low molecular weight heparins. While the choice of anticoagulant as a function of the syndrome is largely outside the realm of this text, the number of breastfeeding mothers exposed to these compounds is significant and warrants coverage. The mechanism of action of these compounds varies enormously. Warfarin is a typical competitive inhibitor of vitamin K-dependent carboxylation of factors II, VII, IX and X and thus depletes the procoagulant factors. Heparin inhibits coagulation by its action on antithrombin III, which is a natural inhibitor of factors XIIa, XIa, Xa, IXa, IIa (thrombin) and plasmin. The low molecular weight heparins (enoxaparin, dalteparin) work similarly but with fewer side effects than heparin. Platelet-inhibitory drugs both reversibly or irreversibly inhibit platelet cyclo-oxygenase thus inhibiting platelet aggregation or synthesis of platelet factors such as thromboxane A2. Aspirin is a typical irreversible antiplatelet medication. Heparin induced thrombocytopenia (HIT) and heparin induced thrombosis (HITTS) are rare complications related to heparin therapy and require discontinuation of heparin and the choice of an alternative anti-coagulant such as argatroban.

ARGATROBAN   **AAP:** Not Reviewed

Trade: Argatroban
Can/Aus/UK:
Specifics: Synthetic, direct thrombin inhibitor which reversibly binds to the thrombin active site. Administered by intravenous continuous infusion, MW=526 daltons. Probably too large to enter milk.
T½= 39-51 min.   Oral= Poor   Peak= 1-3 hours

DIPYRIDAMOLE   **AAP:** Not Reviewed

Trade: Persantine
Can/Aus/UK: Apo-Dipyridamole, Novo-Dipiradol, Persantin
Specifics: Milk levels are believed to be very low. No reported side effects.
T½= 10-12 hours   Oral= Poor   Peak= 45-150 min.
LRC= L3

HEPARIN

AAP: Not Reviewed

Trade: Heparin
Can/Aus/UK:
Specifics: Heparin is a large molecular weight protein (40,000 daltons) that is not secreted into human milk. Further, it is not orally bioavailable.
T½= 1-2 hours   Oral= None   Peak= 20 min.
LRC= L1

WARFARIN

AAP: Compatible

Trade: Coumadin, Panwarfin
Can/Aus/UK: Coumadin, Warfilone, Marevan
Specifics: Warfarin is highly protein bound. Milk levels are virtually undetectable. In numerous studies, no effect on breastfeeding infants have been reported.
T½= 1-2.5 days   Oral= Complete   Peak= 0.5-3 days
LRC= L2

ENOXAPARIN

AAP: Not Reviewed

Trade: Lovenox, Low Molecular Weight Heparin
Can/Aus/UK: Lovenox, Clexane
Specifics: Low molecular fraction (2000-8000 daltons) of heparin. Transfer into human milk is very unlikely due to large molecular weight.
T½= 4.5 hours   Oral= None   Peak= 3-5 hours
LRC= L3

DALTEPARIN SODIUM

AAP: Not Reviewed

Trade: Fragmin, Low Molecular Weight Heparin
Can/Aus/UK:
Specifics: In another study of 15 post-caesarian patients following subcutaneous doses of 2500 IU, maternal plasma levels averaged 0.074 to 0.308 IU/mL. Breastmilk levels of dalteparin ranged from < 0.005 to 0.037 IU/mL of milk. Using this data, an infant ingesting 150 mL/kg/day would ingest approximately 5.5 IU/kg/day. Due to the polysaccharide nature of this production, oral absorption is unlikely. The authors suggested that "It appears highly unlikely that puerperal thromboprophylaxis with LMWH has any clinically relevant effect on the nursing infant".
T½= 2.3 hours   Oral= None   Peak= 2-4 hours (SC)
LRC= L2

TINZAPARIN   AAP: Not Reviewed

Trade: Innohep
Can/Aus/UK: Innohep
Specifics: Tinzaparin is a low molecular weight heparin with antithrombotic properties used for the treatment of deep vein thrombosis. No data are available on its transfer to milk. However, due to its protein nature and its large molecular weight, breastmilk levels would be expected to be quite low. Some breastfeeding data are available for a similar product, dalteparin.

T½= 2.3 hours   Oral= None   Peak= 2-4 hours (SC)
LRC= L3

Clinical Tips:

Warfarin has been extensively used in breastfeeding mothers, and in no cases have they found changes in the breastfed infant's coagulation, nor warfarin levels in the neonate that were clinically relevant. Warfarin is extensively bound to protein in the maternal plasma compartment (> 99%) and does not penetrate into milk to any degree. Several studies have documented its safe use. Heparin is a large molecular weight protein (40,000 daltons) and is unable to penetrate milk. Further, it would not be orally bioavailable in an infant even if it did penetrate milk. The low molecular weight heparins (enoxaparin, dalteparin) are still 2000-9000 daltons in size and are far too large to enter milk in clinically relevant concentrations. They are not orally bioavailable. A new study shows that only minimal amounts of dalteparin are secreted into human milk (5.5 IU/kg/day). However, anticoagulant therapy in breastfeeding mothers should always be approached cautiously with close observation of the infant for signs of abnormal bleeding. The use of antiplatelet medications in breastfeeding mothers is less well understood. While it is true that aspirin and dipyridamole levels in milk have been documented to be very low to undetectable, it is wise to remember that their effect on platelet cyclo-oxygenase is irreversible and requires re-synthesis of the platelet prior to a return of function. For this reason, very small levels of these agents could theoretically alter platelet aggregation to some degree. Some caution with these latter two drugs is advised in breastfeeding situations. The association of aspirin to Reye's syndrome in children is also a possible risk factor but the dose of aspirin via milk is so low that it seems unreasonable to assume it would increase the risk of Reye's syndrome. Secondly, the age of highest incidence of Reye's syndrome is 6 (4-12) years, which is sometimes beyond the breastfeeding period. Another antiplatelet drug, ticlopidine, is even more risky due to severe neutropenia and is only used in those patients who are aspirin intolerant. At this time, without data, ticlopidine would not be a suitable choice for a breastfeeding patient.

Suggested Reading:

1.   Palareti G. A guide to oral anticoagulant therapy. Italian Federation of Anticoagulation Clinics. Haemostasis. 1998;28 Suppl 1:1-46. Review.
2.   Kher A, et al. Laboratory assessment of antithrombotic therapy: what tests and if so

why? Haemostasis. 1997 Sep-Oct;27(5):211-8. Review.

3. Kottkamp H, et al. Role of anticoagulant therapy in atrial fibrillation. J Cardiovasc Electrophysiol. 1998 Aug;9(8Suppl):S86-96. Review.

4. Gibson PS, Rosene-Montella K. Drugs in pregnancy. Anticoagulants. Best Pract Res Clin Obstet Gynaecol 2001; 15(6):847-861.

5. Sullano MA, Ortiz EJ. Deep vein thrombosis and anticoagulant therapy. Nurs Clin North Am 2001; 36(4):645-63.

6. Graham SP. To anticoagulate or not to anticoagulate patients with cardiomyopathy. Cardiol Clin 2001; 19(4):605-615.

7. Cohen M. The role of low-molecular-weight heparin in the management of acute coronary syndromes. Curr Opin Cardiol 2001; 16(6):384-389.

8. Hirsh J, Anand SS, Halperin JL, Fuster V. Guide to anticoagulant therapy: Heparin : a statement for healthcare professionals from the American Heart Association. Circulation 2001; 103(24):2994-3018.

Anxiety Disorders

Principles of Therapy:

Anxiety is apprehension, tension, or uneasiness related to anticipated danger. It may be associated with environmental stress or even devoid of cause. Panic disorder (with or without agoraphobia) is the most common anxiety disorder occurring in 2-6% of the population. When anxiety becomes disproportionate to reality it may become pathologic. Attempts should be made to eliminate other associated diseases such as depression, hyperthyroidism, pheochromocytoma, alcohol use and abuse or psychiatric disorders. There are a number of anxiety disorders which include panic disorders, social phobias, generalized anxiety disorders, obsessive-compulsive disorders, post-traumatic stress disorders, and others.

ALPRAZOLAM   AAP: Not Reviewed

Trade: Xanax
Can/Aus/UK: Apo-Alpraz, Novo-Alprazol, Xanax, Kalma, Ralozam
Specifics: No breastfeeding data is available on this medication except the report of mild withdrawal symptoms in an infant after 9 months of exposure via breastmilk.
T½= 12-15 hours   Oral= Complete   Peak= 1-2 hours
LRC= L3

BUSPIRONE   AAP: Not Reviewed

Trade: BuSpar
Can/Aus/UK: BuSpar, Apo-Buspirone, Novo-Buspirone
Specifics: In many respects Buspirone would appear to be an ideal candidate anxiolytic even though we do not have information on levels in breastmilk. It has a rather short half-life (3 hours) and produces minimal sedation and addiction. However, onset is delayed up to 2 weeks and may not be useful for acute anxiety attacks.
T½= 2-3 hours   Oral= 90%   Peak= 60-90 minutes
LRC= L3

CLOMIPRAMINE   AAP: Compatible

Trade: Anafranil
Can/Aus/UK: Anafranil, Apo-Clomipramine, Placil
Specifics: May be especially useful for panic disorders, or obsessive-compulsive disorder.
T½= 19-37 hours   Oral= Complete   Peak= N/A
LRC= L2

CLONAZEPAM
AAP: Not Reviewed

Trade: Klonopin
Can/Aus/UK: Rivotril, Apo-Clonazepam, PMS-Clonazepam, Paxam
Specifics: Reported milk levels are low, 11-13 µg/L of milk.
T½= 18-50 hours   Oral= Complete   Peak= 1-4 hours
LRC= L3

FLUOXETINE
AAP: May be of concern

Trade: Prozac
Can/Aus/UK: Prozac, Apo-Fluoxetine, Novo-Fluoxetine, Lovan, Zactin
Specifics: Fluoxetine, and its metabolite norfluoxetine have very long half-lives. Several reports indicate high plasma levels in some infants. Symptoms reported include colic, insomnia, tremors, crying, and one case of coma. Use during pregnancy, followed by use during lactation may be inadvisable. Do not use in premature or newborns infants. Its use in older infants (> 4 months) may be less risky.
T½= 2-3 days(fluoxetine)   Oral= 100%   Peak= 1.5 - 12 hours
LRC= L2 in older infants
         L3 if used in neonatal period

IMIPRAMINE
AAP: May be of concern

Trade: Tofranil, Janimine
Can/Aus/UK: Apo-Imipramine, Impril, Novo-Pramine, Melipramine, Tofranil
Specifics: Dose via milk is low and is estimated to be from 20-200 µg per day. No untoward effects noted in breastfed infants.
T½= 8-16 hours   Oral= 90%   Peak= 1-2 hours
LRC= L2

LORAZEPAM
AAP: May be of concern

Trade: Ativan
Can/Aus/UK: Apo-Lorazepam, Ativan, Novo-Lorazepam, Almazine
Specifics: Multiple studies show milk levels of 8-12 µg/L. These are probably too low to produce untoward effects in normal breastfed infants. Long-term use is not recommended.
T½= 12 hours   Oral= 90%   Peak= 2 hours
LRC= L3

MOCLOBEMIDE

AAP: Not Reviewed

Trade:
Can/Aus/UK: Apo-Moclobemide, Arima, Aurorix, Manerix
Specifics: Unlike older MAO inhibitors, moclobemide is a selective and reversible inhibitor of MAO-A isozyme and thus is not plagued with the dangerous side effects of the older MAO inhibitor families. It is an effective treatment for depression. In a study by Pons in 6 lactating women, who received a single oral dose of 300mg, the concentration of moclobemide (Cmax) was highest at 3 hours after the dose and averaged 2.7 mg/L. The average (AUC) milk concentration through the 12 hour period was 0.97 mg/L hour. According to the authors, an average 3.5 kg breastfed infant would therefore be exposed to only a 0.05 mg/kg dose, which is approximately 1% of the maternal dose on a weight basis. The minimal levels of moclobemide found in milk are unlikely to produce untoward effects according to the authors.
T½= 1-2.2 hours   Oral= 80%   Peak= 2 hours
LCR= L3

FLUVOXAMINE

AAP: Not Reviewed

Trade: Luvox
Can/Aus/UK: Luvox, Apo-Fluvoxamine, Alti-Fluvoxamine, Luvox, Faverin, Floxyfral, Myroxim
Specifics: In a case report of one 23 year old mother and following a dose of 100 mg twice daily for 2 weeks, the maternal plasma level of fluvoxamine base was 0.31 mg/Liter and the milk concentration was 0.09 mg/Liter. The authors reported a theoretical dose to infant of 0.0104 mg/kg/day of fluvoxamine, which is only 0.5% of the maternal dose.
T½= 15.6 hours   Oral= 53%   Peak= 3-8 hours
LRC= L2

PAROXETINE

AAP: Not Reviewed

Trade: Paxil
Can/Aus/UK: Paxil, Aropax 20, Seroxat
Specifics: In a recent study of 16 mothers by Stowe, paroxetine levels in milk were low and varied according to maternal dose. Milk/plasma ratios varied from 0.056 to 1.3. Milk levels ranged from approximately 17 µg/L, 45 µg/L, 70 µg/L, 92 µg/L, and 101 µg/L in mothers receiving a dose of 10, 20, 30, 40, and 50 mg/day respectively. Levels of paroxetine were below the limit of detection (< 2 ng/mL) in all 16 infants. Numerous other studies generally conclude that paroxetine can be considered relatively safe for breastfeeding infants as the absolute dose transferred is quite low. Plasma levels in the infant were generally undetectable. Recent data suggests that a

neonatal withdrawal syndrome may occur in newborns exposed in utero to paroxetine.

T½= 21 hours   Oral= Complete   Peak= 5-8 hours
LRC= L2

PROPRANOLOL   AAP: Compatible

Trade: Inderal
Can/Aus/UK: Detensol, Inderal, Novo-Pranol, Deralin, Cardinol
Specifics: Propranolol is an ideal beta-blocker for breastfeeding women. Numerous studies show minimal milk levels and minimal to no side effects in the infant.

T½= 3-5 hours   Oral= 30%   Peak= 60-90 min.
LRC= L3

SERTRALINE   AAP: Not Reviewed

Trade: Zoloft
Can/Aus/UK: Zoloft, Lustral
Specifics: At this time, more than 60 breastfeeding infants have been studied following maternal use of sertraline. Thus far, no untoward effects have been reported, and in almost all cases, only subclinical levels of sertraline was detectable in the plasma compartment of the infant.

T½= 26-65 hours   Oral= Complete   Peak= 7-8 hours
LRC= L2

TRAZODONE   AAP: May be of concern

Trade: Desyrel
Can/Aus/UK:
Specifics: In six mothers who received a single 50 mg dose, the milk/plasma ratio averaged 0.14.   Peak milk concentrations occurred at 2 hours   On a weight basis, an adult would receive 0.77 mg/kg whereas a breastfeeding infant, using this data, would consume only 0.005 mg/kg. About 0.6 % of the maternal dose was ingested by the infant.

T½= 4-9 hours   Oral= 65%   Peak= 1-2 hours
LRC= L2

VENLAFAXINE   AAP: Not Reviewed

Trade: Effexor
Can/Aus/UK: Effexor
Specifics: The mean total infant dose was 7.6% of the maternal weight-adjusted dose. The metabolite of venlafaxine (but not venlafaxine) was detected in all three infants at low levels. The infants were healthy and showed

no acute adverse effects.
T½= 5 hours(venlafaxine)   Oral= 92%   Peak= N/A
LRC= L3

Clinical Tips:
Panic Disorder:
The psychopharmacological treatment of panic disorders has changed dramatically in the past few years.   Previously, benzodiazepines were typical first line therapy while today the antidepressants especially the serotonin reuptake inhibitors (SSRIs), have become first-line therapy in many patients.   Of the antidepressants, imipramine has been used and studied the longest.   One large study of imipramine and alprazolam in 1168 patients found that they were equally effective, and both drugs were superior to placebo.   Imipramine should be started at low doses (25-50 mg) and increased gradually.   Most patients achieve relief at 150-250 mg/day.   However, milk levels of imipramine are generally higher than other tricyclic antidepressants and some concern over its use is recommended.   About 25% of patients with panic disorder report a 'jitteriness syndrome' with imipramine;   doses should be reduced to relieve this symptom.   Clomipramine, amitriptyline, and nortriptyline have been found useful but fewer studies are available attesting to their efficacy.   Trazodone has been found to be less useful although its milk levels are low.   Limited data also suggests venlafaxine may be useful in panic disorder.

The preferred SSRIs are fluoxetine, paroxetine, fluvoxamine, sertraline, and clomipramine as these have been found to be very effective.   Patients sometimes report a 'jitteriness syndrome' consisting of restlessness, sweating, flushing, or even increase anxiety.   To avoid this response, many clinicians begin therapy with one-quarter to one-half the usual therapeutic dose and gently increase as tolerated.   Low doses of benzodiazepines such as alprazolam can be used temporarily to counteract this symptom.   Because the SSRIs can induce manic symptoms in some patients, a careful family history of bipolar disorder should be obtained.

The benzodiazepines are known to be effective treatment for phobic disorder, panic attacks, and anticipatory anxiety.   Several large studies of alprazolam found it clinically effective in reducing panic attacks.   Diazepam, while effective, requires much larger doses (20-60 mg) which may be sedating.   These doses would not be ideal for a breastfeeding mother as diazepam has a long half-life and measurable milk levels.   While alprazolam is more potent and effective than diazepam, it also suffers from a shorter half-life thus requiring more frequent dosing or the use of a sustained-release product.   Effective doses of alprazolam vary enormously between patients but should be initiated at 0.25 to 0.5 mg three times daily and then increased as symptoms require.   The undesirable effects of benzodiazepines include sedation, potentiation of alcohol, dependence, and significant withdrawal effects.   Withdrawal can be severe and should be carried out over many days to weeks.   Withdrawal symptoms include profound insomnia, anxiety, panic, tremor, and depersonalization.

The presence of insomnia (which primarily only occurs in withdrawal) is a major means of differentiating between withdrawal and the return of anxiety symptoms. Because of the withdrawal effects, many patients refuse to stop benzodiazepines. Interestingly, in one breastfeeding mother who did withdraw, her breastfed infant subsequently exhibited withdrawal symptoms.

As a family, the benzodiazepines tend to have rather long half-lives and could potentially (after prolonged administration) build up in the plasma compartment of the breastfed infant although this has not been reported. This could lead to sedation and increased risk of apnea. Therefore, recommend the shorter half-life medications such as alprazolam or lorazepam if a benzodiazepine is required. Use cautiously in premature infants or those subject to apnea. Remember, short intervals of use (24-72 hours) are less risky than long term therapy, especially with the longer half-life products like diazepam. We have no data on buspirone in breastmilk, but its unique lack of sedation or addiction may be useful in breastfeeding situations. However, while it may be effective for anxiety disorders, it is ineffective for panic disorder.

Anxiety Disorder:
The main features of anxiety disorder are chronic, behavioral, and physiological symptoms of anxiety and hyperarousal. Because anxiety disorders often coexist with depression and panic disorders, in this situation, depression and panic should be initially treated as above. The treatment of anxiety disorders in the past has mainly required the use of the benzodiazepines, but newer data suggests that imipramine, venlafaxine, and clomipramine may be quite effective as well. Buspirone has been found as effective as the benzodiazepines in some studies although this is not always seen clinically. At present we do not have data on breastmilk levels of buspirone, however, it produces less drowsiness, psychomotor impairment, alcohol potentiation, and far less addiction than the benzodiazepines in patients, and it is probably a good candidate for breastfeeding mothers even without clear milk levels. Doses of buspirone average 20-40 mg/day and it is clearly effective for the anxious patient and also to lessen the withdrawal following use of the benzodiazepines. Regardless, it should not be used solely for withdrawal but in combination with declining doses of the benzodiazepine.

Obsessive-Compulsive Disorders:
Treatment of this disorder is not that different from other anxiety disorders. Clomipramine, fluoxetine, fluvoxamine, paroxetine, and sertraline have been found to be effective and should be considered first line therapy although many patients still suffer from symptoms to some degree. While clomipramine and the SSRIs are apparently equally efficacious, the side effect profile of clomipramine is somewhat troublesome for some patients and includes anticholinergic effects (blurred vision, constipation, and dry mouth), sedation, and toxicity in overdose which is also common with the tricyclic antidepressants. Prior studies suggest therapy of at least 6 weeks is required at doses up to 300 mg/d to alleviate symptoms. Therapy with the

SSRIs, particularly fluvoxamine and fluoxetine, have been found equally effective although they too require up to 4-6 weeks of therapy; 10-12 weeks of therapy are required prior to assuming these medication are ineffective. Doses are less clear. Some studies have found that 20 mg/d of fluoxetine is just as effective as 40-60 mg/d. Doses should probably be increased gently over time to affect therapy. Clinical efficacy of various medications should not be discounted until the patient has been treated with a minimum daily dose of the following : clomipramine 250mg, fluoxetine 60 mg, fluvoxamine 300 mg, paroxetine 60 mg, and sertraline 200 mg. In breastfeeding patients with young infants, the above higher doses could prove problematic, particularly with fluoxetine and clomipramine. Caution is recommended at the higher doses in breastfeeding mothers early postpartum. The use of neuroleptics is controversial. Although some patients may respond positively, numerous case reports of worsening symptoms can be found, particularly with risperidone and clozapine.

Social Phobia:
While social phobia may share several features with panic disorder, it has several unique phenomenologic features. The five most common fears of patients with social phobias are: 1) public speaking, 2) eating in public, 3) using public lavatories, 4) writing in public, 5) being the object of attention. Shyness and avoidance are typical features of this syndrome. Paroxetine and fluvoxamine have been found to be very effective for these symptoms although other SSRIs may be used such as fluoxetine and sertraline. The monamine oxidase inhibitors are also effective. However, we do not recommend their use in the USA as our MAOI drugs are irreversible inhibitors and overtime could produce significant MAO inhibition in breastfed infants (undocumented). Other countries use the newer reversible MAOi drugs which may be safer (see Moclobemide) although one study did not find moclobemide better than placebo. Other medications that have been found to be effective include the benzodiazepines, alprazolam, and clonazepam. Gabapentin also appears to be effective in the disorder although its use in breastfeeding mothers has not been published (unpublished data by the author suggests milks levels are low).

Suggested Reading:

1. Roy-Byrne PP, et al. Search for pathophysiology of panic disorder. Lancet. 1998 Nov 21;352(9141):1646-7. Review.
2. Amin MM, Ban TA, Pecknold JC, Klingner A. Clomipramine (Anafranil) and behaviour therapy in obsessive-compulsive and phobic disorders. J Int Med Res. 1977;5 Suppl 5:33-7.
3. Sansone RA, et al. Panic disorder: the ultimate anxiety. J Womens Health. 1998 Oct;7(8):983-9. Review.
4. Davidson JR. Pharmacotherapy of social anxiety disorder. J Clin Psychiatry. 1998;59 Suppl 17:47-53. Review.
5. Barlow DH, et al. DSM-IV and beyond: what is generalized anxiety disorder? Acta Psychiatr Scand Suppl. 1998;393:23-9. Review.

Asthma

Principles of Therapy:

Asthma is defined as a chronic inflammatory disorder of the airways in which many cells play a role, particularly mast cells, eosinophils, and T lymphocytes. Most asthmatics are atopic. Symptoms vary from recurrent episodes of wheezing, breathlessness, and cough to severe respiratory distress. Increasingly, in the last decade, asthma has become recognized as an inflammatory process of the bronchi requiring anti-inflammatory treatment early on in the process. Initially, treatment consists of removal of offending allergens such as cigarette smoke, animal dander, dust mites, and more recently, cockroaches. Early therapeutic intervention is presently aimed at controlling the inflammatory process. Presently, mast cell stabilizing agents (e.g. cromolyn and nedocromil) and inhaled synthetic corticosteroids should be considered for first line therapy. Adjuncts to therapy also include the selective beta-2 agonists (e.g. albuterol, terbutaline, salmeterol) which provide relief of acute bronchoconstriction. The older beta agonist, isoproterenol, should not be used in asthmatics today. The anticholinergic agent ipratropium is useful in reflex cholinergic bronchoconstriction, particularly from cold air-induced asthma, sulfur dioxide-induced asthma, and cough-variant asthma. Theophylline is only occasionally used today, as it is a moderate to poor bronchodilator, and it has a number of unwelcome side effects (arrhythmias). The newer leukotriene inhibitors (e.g. zafirlukast, montelukast), when used prophylactically, are useful in some patients in reducing the inflammatory response, but studies are inconclusive as to their overall usefulness.

ALBUTEROL   **AAP:** Not Reviewed

> **Trade:** Proventil, Ventolin
> **Can/Aus/UK:** Novo-Salmol, Ventolin, Asmavent, Respax,Respolin, Asmol, Salbulin, Salbuvent
> **Specifics:** Less than 10% of inhaled albuterol is systemically absorbed. This would not likely produce clinically relevant levels in breastfed infants. In addition, the dose of albuterol on a mg/kg basis is higher in infants than in adults.
> T½= 3.8 hours   Oral= 100%   Peak= 5-30 min.
> LRC= L1

BECLOMETHASONE   **AAP:** Not Reviewed

> **Trade:** Vanceril, Beclovent
> **Can/Aus/UK:** Propaderm, Vanceril, Beconase, Becloforte, Aldecin, Becotide, Beclovent, Propadem
> **Specifics:** Intrapulmonary doses are exceedingly low and penetration into

47

milk is extremely remote. Maternal plasma levels are virtually undetectable.

T½= 15 hours   Oral= 90%   Peak= N/A
LRC= L2

CROMOLYN SODIUM   AAP: Not Reviewed

Trade: Intal
Can/Aus/UK: Intral
Specifics: Cromolyn is not systemically absorbed by the mother nor infant.
It would not be orally bioavailable by the infant. It is virtually nontoxic.
T½= 80-90 minutes   Oral= < 1%   Peak= < 15 minutes
LRC= L1

FLUNISOLIDE   AAP: Not Reviewed

Trade: AeroBid
Can/Aus/UK:
Specifics: Systemic absorption of intrapulmonary doses is exceedingly low
(< 40%). Transfer of clinically relevant amounts in milk is very remote.
T½= 1.8 hours   Oral= 21%   Peak= 30 min.
LRC= L3

FLUTICASONE   AAP: Not Reviewed

Trade: Flovent
Can/Aus/UK: Flovent
Specifics: Oral and topical absorption of fluticasone is less than 2%, so it is
virtually unabsorbed. Transfer into milk is remote. Currently available for
use in infants.
T½= 7.8 hours   Oral= <2%   Peak= 15-60 min.
LRC= L3

LEVALBUTEROL   AAP: Not Reviewed

Trade: Xopenex
Can/Aus/UK: Xopenex
Specifics: Levalbuterol is the active (R)-enantiomer of the drug substance
racemic albuterol.   No data are available on breastmilk levels.   After
inhalation, plasma levels are incredibly low, averaging 1.1 nanogram/mL.   It
is very unlikely that enough would enter milk to produce clinical effects in an
infant.   This product is commonly used in infancy for asthma and other
bronchoconstrictive illnesses.
T½= 3.3 hours   Oral= N/A   Peak= 0.2 hours
LRC= L2

NEDOCROMIL SODIUM
AAP: Not Reviewed

Trade: Tilade
Can/Aus/UK: Tilade, Mireze
Specifics: Poor oral bioavailability and limited toxicity of this compound would produce minimal problems for a breastfed infant.
T½= 3.3 hours   Oral= 8-17%   Peak= 28 min.
LRC= L2

SALMETEROL XINAFOATE
AAP: Not Reviewed

Trade: Serevent
Can/Aus/UK: Serevent
Specifics: Salmeterol use in breastfeeding mothers has not been reported, but its systemic absorption in the mother would be incredibly small due to sequestration in the bronchial tissue. Adult plasma levels are virtually undetectable.
T½= 5.5 hours   Oral= Complete   Peak= 10 - 45 min.
LRC= L2

TERBUTALINE
AAP: Compatible

Trade: Bricanyl, Brethine
Can/Aus/UK: Bricanyl
Specifics: Following the oral administration in mothers, milk levels were minimal. No untoward effects were noted in breastfed infants.
T½= 14 hours   Oral= 33-50%   Peak= 5-30 min.
LRC= L2

THEOPHYLLINE
AAP: Compatible

Trade: Aminophylline, Quibron, Theo-dur
Can/Aus/UK: Theo-Dur, Pulmophylline, Quibron-T/SR, Austyn, Nuelin
Specifics: Milk levels are low. Estimated dose absorbed by infant is approximately 1% of maternal dose.
T½= 3-12.8 hours   Oral= 76%   Peak= 1-2 hours
LRC= L3

TRIAMCINOLONE ACETONIDE
AAP: Not Reviewed

Trade: Azmacort
Can/Aus/UK: Azmacort
Specifics: Intrapulmonary doses of triamcinolone are exceedingly small and are extremely unlikely to produce clinically relevant levels in human milk. Intra-articular doses, due to slow absorption, would not be likely to produce

high milk levels.
T½= 88 minutes   Oral= Complete   Peak= N/A
LRC= L3

ZAFIRLUKAST   **AAP:** Not Reviewed

Trade: Accolate
Can/Aus/UK:
Specifics: Zafirlukast transfer into human milk is extremely low (< 50 n/mL). Further, it is poorly bioavailable when administered with food. It is unlikely to produce side effects in an infant.
T½= 10-13 hours   Oral= Poor   Peak= 3 hours
LRC= L3

BUDESONIDE   **AAP:** Not Reviewed

Trade: Rhinocort, Pulmocort
Can/Aus/UK:
Specifics: Budesonide is weakly bioavailable (<20%), and it is a weak systemic corticosteroid. It is very unlikely to penetrate milk nor cause systemic effects in the infant.
T½= 2.8 hours   Oral= 10.7%   Peak= 2-4 hours
LRC= L3

METHYLPREDNISOLONE   **AAP:** Compatible

Trade: Solu-Medrol, Depo-Medrol, Medrol
Can/Aus/UK:
Specifics: Transfer of methylprednisolone into milk has not been studied, but studies of rather high doses of prednisone(120 mg/day) find only minimal, subclinical transfer. See prednisone.
T½= 2.8 hours   Oral= Complete   Peak= N/A
LRC= L2

Clinical Tips: The goals of asthma therapy are to prevent bronchoconstriction, expiratory wheezing, maintenance of normal lung function, a normal quality of life, and to minimize pharmacologic side effects. In general, asthma is classified by the severity and frequency of attacks. Varying from mild episodic, to mild persistent, to moderate persistent and finally, severe persistent attacks. Treatment is dependent on the classification within which the patient fits. In the last decade more emphasis has been placed on treating the etiology of bronchoconstriction, namely inflammation, particularly using more inhaled steroids. In the patient with mild episodic asthma, broncho dilators such as albuterol are indicated. As the severity of attacks increase, the use of inhaled corticosteroids along with long-acting beta agonists (salmeterol) has become the mainstay of treatment. The use of higher and higher doses of inhaled corticosteroids, such as fluticasone and budesonide, has become standard therapy.

In breastfeeding mothers, the mast-cell stabilizers (e.g. cromolyn and nedocromil) are some of the safest drugs one can use in asthmatics. They are not orally bioavailable and would not penetrate milk at all. However, they are not very efficacious and are seldom used today.

The most commonly used medications, albuterol and salmeterol, are poorly absorbed from the pulmonary mucosa. Less than 21-30% of albuterol is absorbed into the plasma compartment following administration via inhalation. Even then, peak plasma levels are in the low nanogram range. While not known, it is likely milk levels would be so low as to be undetectable. Levalbuterol (Xopenex) is the active R-isomer of albuterol and its milk kinetics would be similar to albuterol. Salmeterol has a high binding affinity for lung tissue and is retained for many hours prior to elimination. These products have been used extensively in breastfeeding mothers without reported side effect in their infants.

The inhaled corticosteroids, particularly fluticasone and budesonide, are administered in microgram quantities. Because of poor bioavailability, plasma steroid levels in most asthmatics following intrapulmonary use is extremely low. Although we do not have breastmilk studies, the incredibly low plasma levels would obviously produce even lower levels in milk. Hence, it is unlikely the small amount penetrating milk would be clinically relevant to a breastfed infant as the oral bioavailability of these products are very low (ranging 1-10%). Thus far, no untoward effects on breastfed infants have been reported when exposed via milk. Of this family, fluticasone would appear to have the best kinetics (< 1% oral bioavailability) for breastfeeding mothers and their infants. The short-term use of oral or IV corticosteroids is not necessarily contraindicated because steroids have been documented to penetrate milk poorly. Even high oral doses of prednisone (120 mg daily) do not produce clinically relevant levels in milk. Short-term therapy with high doses would not likely affect a breastfed infant.

Of the leukotriene inhibitors, only Zafirlukast has been studied in breastfeeding mothers. Following repeated 40 mg doses twice daily, the average steady-state concentration in breastmilk was only 50 µg/L compared to 255 ng/mL in maternal plasma. Zafirlukast is poorly absorbed when administered with food. It is likely the oral absorption via ingestion of breastmilk would be low. Other leukotriene inhibitors such as montelukast(Singulair) have not been studied.

Suggested Reading:

1. Kemp JP. Comprehensive asthma management: guidelines for clinicians. J Asthma. 1998;35(8):601-20. Review.
2. Gross KM, et al. New strategies in the medical management of asthma. Am Fam

Physician. 1998 Jul;58(1):89-100, 109-12. Review.

3. Bone RC. Goals of asthma management. A step-care approach. Chest. 1996 Apr;109(4):1056-65. Review.

4. Keenan JM. Asthma management. The case for aiming at control rather than merely relief. Postgrad Med. 1998 Mar;103(3):53-9, 62-5, 69. Review.

5. Cockcroft DW, et al. Outpatient asthma management. Med Clin North Am. 1996 Jul;80(4):701-18. Review.

6. Naureckas ET, Solway J. Clinical practice. Mild asthma. N Engl J Med. 2001 Oct 25;345(17):1257-62. Review.

7. Kips JC, Pauwels RA. Long-acting inhaled beta(2)-agonist therapy in asthma. Am J Respir Crit Care Med. 2001 Sep 15;164(6):923-32. Review.

8. Hunt LW. How to manage difficult asthma cases. An action plan for physicians and patients. Postgrad Med. 2001 May;109(5):61-8. Review.

9. Expert Panel Report 2 Guidelines for Diagnosis and Management of Asthma, National Institute of Health, National Heart Lung, and Blood Institute, 1997.

Atopic Dermatitis

Principles of Therapy:

Atopic dermatitis is a chronic, severely pruritic skin disorder characterized by dry skin, eczematous patches, and thickening of the skin. Diagnostic criteria must generally include pruritus, weepy, shiny, or lichenified patches, and a tendency toward chronic or relapsing dermatitis. Patients frequently have elevated antibody levels (IgE) and a family or personal history of other allergic diseases such as allergic rhinitis or asthma. Exacerbating factors in atopic dermatitis include dry skin, sensitivity to irritants (e.g. wool, sweat, saliva, foods, chemicals), infection (*Staph Aureus*), and stress. The distribution of lesions is characteristic, with involvement of the face, neck, and trunk. Elbows and knees are typically involved as well. Adult lesions are usually dry, leathery, hyperpigmented, or hypopigmented (particularly in black patients). Treatment includes removal of stress or irritating factors, less frequent bathing (brief and with mild soaps) followed by application of emollients or lotions, humidification of the home environment (during dry winters), mild topical corticosteroids, antipruritics (e.g. hydroxyzine, diphenhydramine), and topical or oral antibacterial preparations.

DIPHENHYDRAMINE   AAP: Not Reviewed

Trade: Benadryl, Cheracol
Can/Aus/UK: Allerdryl, Benadryl, Insomnal, Nytol, Delixir, Paedamin
Specifics: Diphenhydramine is a short-acting but effective antihistamine. Sedation is the most common side effect. There are suggestions that milk supply may be suppressed but these are unsubstantiated. Nevertheless, some caution is due.

T½= 4.3 hours   Oral= 43-61%   Peak= 2-3 hours
LRC= L2

FLUTICASONE TOPICAL   AAP: Not Reviewed

Trade: Cutivate
Can/Aus/UK:
Specifics: Fluticasone is a medium-potency topical corticosteroid. However, topical fluticasone is poorly absorbed transcutaneously and even less absorbed orally (<1%). Although expensive, it would be an ideal product for use in breastfeeding mothers, especially for large area use.

T½= 7.8 hours   Oral= <1 %   Peak= N/A
LRC= L3

HYDROCORTISONE TOPICAL   **AAP:** Not Reviewed

Trade: Westcort
Can/Aus/UK: Cortate, Cortone, Emo-Cort, Aquacort, Dermaid, Egocort, Hycor, Cortef, Dermacort
Specifics: Topical hydrocortisone is relatively impotent and may require several days to work. Absorption in the infant is minimal.
T½= 1-2 hours   Oral= 96%   Peak= N/A
LRC= L2

HYDROXYZINE   **AAP:** Not Reviewed

Trade: Atarax, Vistaril
Can/Aus/UK: Apo-Hydroxyzine, Atarax, Novo-Hydroxyzin
Specifics: Milk levels are unreported, but it has been safely used for years in pediatric patients.
T½= 3-7 hours   Oral= Complete   Peak= 2 hours
LRC= L1

MUPIROCIN OINTMENT   **AAP:** Not Reviewed

Trade: Bactroban
Can/Aus/UK: Bactroban
Specifics: Topical antibacterial effective for staph, and strep infections. No absorption from topical application.
T½= 17-36 min.   Oral= Complete   Peak= N/A
LRC= L1

TRIAMCINOLONE ACETONIDE   **AAP:** Not Reviewed

Trade: Flutex, Kenalog, Aristocort
Can/Aus/UK: Aristocort, Kenalog, Triaderm, Kenalone, Adcortyl
Specifics: Triamcinolone is considered a moderately potent steroid. Percutaneous absorption is minimal. It is unlikely that systemic absorption by a breastfeeding infant would be significant. Limit amount applied to a minimum.
T½= 88 minutes   Oral= Complete   Peak= N/A
LRC= L3

MOMETASONE   **AAP:** Not Reviewed

Trade: Elocon Ointment
Can/Aus/UK:
Specifics: Topical mometasone is a medium potency steroid. Transfer to milk is unreported and probably minimal. Mometasone is considered a

moderate potency topical steroid.

T½= N/A   Oral= N/A   Peak= N/A
LRC= L3

TACROLIMUS   AAP: Not Reviewed

Trade: Prograf, Protopic
Can/Aus/UK: Protopic
Specifics: Tacrolimus is an immunosuppressant formerly known as SK506. In one report of 21 mothers who received tacroliumus while pregnant, milk concentrations in colostrum averaged 0.79 ng/mL and varied from 0.3 to 1.9 nanograms/mL.   Using this data and an average daily milk intake of 150 mL/kg, the average dose to the infant per day via milk would be < 0.1 µg/kg/day. Because the oral bioavailability is poor (<32%), an infant would likely ingest less than 100 ng/kg/day.   Recently, the FDA approved a topical form of tacrolimus (Protopic) for use in moderate to severe eczema in those for whom standard eczema therapies are deemed inadvisable. Transcutaneous absorption is minimal. In a study of 46 adult patients after multiple doses, plasma levels ranged from undetectable to 20 ng/mL, with 45 of the patients having peak blood concentrations less than 5 ng/mL.   In another study, the peak blood levels averaged 1.6 ng/mL, which is significantly less than the therapeutic range in kidney transplantation(7-20 ng/mL). While the absolute transcutaneous bioavailability is unknown it is apparently very low. Combined with the poor oral bioavailability of this product it is not likely a breastfed infant will receive enough following topical use

T½= 34.2 hours   Oral= 14-32%   Peak=1.6 hours
LRC= L3

Clinical Tips:

Therapy of atopic dermatitis begins with education of the patient and includes instruction on reducing bathing and use of lubricants on the skin. Long showers, harsh detergents, shower brushes, and bubble baths should be avoided although daily bathing is still recommended depending on the climate. Bathing hydrates the stratum corneum and removes bacteria, but the application of a lubricant must be applied within 3 minutes to seal the moisture in the skin.   Moisturizers of choice include: Eucerin, Moisturel, Curel, Complex 15 creams or lotions. Avoid Vaseline intensive Care lotion. Pure Vaseline, Aquaphor, and Crisco are back in fashion but may be a bit heavy in some instances.

Topical steroids, particularly ointments (avoid lotions, gels), are preferred short-term therapy.   Low to medium potency steroids are preferred (e.g. hydrocortisone, triamcinolone, mometasone, fluticasone). High potency steroids should be avoided. Hydroxyzine is the antihistamine/antipruritic of choice although it induces significant sedation. Although we have no data on hydroxyzine transfer to milk, it is a commonly used pediatric antihistamine. Diphenhydramine is an effective antihistamine/antipruritic as well but if used consistently could potentially produce sedation and/or hallucinations in the breastfed infant. As antipruritics, the antihistamines work poorly and only those associated with significant sedation seem effective. Hydroxyzine and cetirizine (Zyrtec) are the effective. Doxepin is an effective antipruritic, but one report of dangerous sedation and apnea in a breastfeeding infant suggests that it may not be suitable for breastfeeding mothers.

The most common complication of atopic dermatitis is super-infection with *Staphylococcus aureus*. Topical neomycin and lanolin are allergic triggers and should be avoided. Mupirocin ointment would be an ideal choice for staphylococcus or streptococcus infections. For severe infections, anti-staphylococcal systemic medications are required and could include Amoxicillin + clavulanate (Augmentin), cephalexin, cloxacillin, and others depending on sensitivity.

Since patients with atopic dermatitis have defects in cell-mediated immunity, the immunosuppressant macrolides (cyclosporine and tacrolimus) may prove to be beneficial in the treatment of this syndrome. Topical tacrolimus has been frequently studied in the treatment of atopic dermatitis because it was found to have better skin penetration and higher potency than topically applied cyclosporine. Numerous studies evaluating the use of topical tacrolimus are available and provide evidence that topical tacrolimus is effective in the treatment of this syndrome with no evidence thus far of systemic adverse effects. The FDA has approved a topical form of tacrolimus (Protopic) for use in moderate to severe eczema, in those for whom standard eczema therapies are deemed inadvisable because of potential risks. Absorption via skin is minimal. In a study of 46 adult patients after multiple doses, plasma levels ranged from undetectable to 20 ng/mL with 45 of the patients having peak blood concentrations less than 5 ng/mL. In another study, the peak blood levels averaged 1.6 ng/mL which is significantly less than the therapeutic range in kidney transplantation(7-20 ng/mL). While the absolute transcutaneous bioavailability is unknown, it is apparently very low (< 0.5%). Combined with the poor oral bioavailability of this product, it is not likely a breastfed infant will receive enough following topical use (maternal) to produce adverse effects.

Suggested Reading:

1. Reynolds NJ. Recent advances in atopic dermatitis. J R Coll Physicians Lond. 1997 May-Jun;31(3):241-5. Review.
2. Graham-Brown RA. Therapeutics in atopic dermatitis. Adv Dermatol. 1997;13:3-31. Review.
3. Rudikoff D, et al. Atopic dermatitis. Lancet. 1998 Jun 6;351(9117):1715-21. Review.
4. Jain A, Venkataramanan R, et.al. Pregnancy after liver transplantation under tacrolimus. Transplantation 64(4):559-565.
5. Gianni LM, Sulli MM. Topical tacrolimus in the treatment of atopic dermatitis. Ann Pharmacother. 2001 Jul-Aug;35(7-8):943-6. Review.

6. Nasr IS. Topical tacrolimus in dermatology. Clin Exp Dermatol. 2000 May;25(3):250-4. Review.
7. http://pedeczema.com/
8. http://www.niams.nih.gov/hi/topics/dermatitis/

Bipolar Disorder - Mania

Principles of Therapy:

The essential feature of Bipolar disorder is the presence of chronic depression and occasional episodes of mania. Mania is characterized by inflated self esteem or grandiosity, elation with hyperactivity, flight of ideas, over enthusiasm, easy distractability, and insomnia. Compared with unipolar depression, the depressive phase of bipolar disorder includes symptoms such as hypersomnia, hyperphagia and weight gain, and decreased energy. Approximately one-half of all bipolar patients also have psychotic symptoms. Psychotic symptomatology is reduced more in divalproex-treated than in lithium-treated patients. The mainstay of treatment of mania has been lithium, although acute episodes may require neuroleptics such as haloperidol(Haldol) or clonazepam. Although lithium use in breastfeeding mothers is controversial, some recent studies suggest that with close observation, lithium levels in the neonate are usually subclinical. More recently, the use of valproic acid, clozapine, and carbamazepine have been found to be effective alternatives to those who refuse or cannot take lithium. Bipolar disorder is strongly associated with several other disorders: migraine, obsessive-compulsive disorder, panic disorder, and attention-deficit/hyperactivity disorder. Valproic acid, because of its efficacy in treating migraine, mania, panic, and OCD, has assumed a more important role in the therapy of this disorder particularly with the presence of the above comorbid conditions and in mania associated with substance abuse. Manic patients with mixed depressive symptoms respond less to lithium than those with pure or elated mania. Patients with coincident substance abuse, respond less to lithium, and better to valproate treatment.

BUPROPION   AAP: Not Reviewed

Trade: Wellbutrin, Zyban
Can/Aus/UK:
Specifics: While this drug has a high milk/plasma ratio, it is not detectable in the infants plasma. Hence the absolute dose via milk is very low. May lower seizure threshold. Do not use in patients subject to seizures.
T½= 8-24 hours   Oral= N/A   Peak= 2 hours
LRC= L3

CLOMIPRAMINE   AAP: Compatible

Trade: Anafranil
Can/Aus/UK: Anafranil, Apo-Clomipramine, Placil
Specifics: May be especially useful for panic disorders, or obsessive-compulsive disorder.

T½= 19-37 hours   Oral= Complete   Peak= N/A
LRC= L2

DESIPRAMINE   AAP: May be of concern

Trade: Pertofrane, Norpramin
Can/Aus/UK: Norpramin, Pertofrane, Novo-Desipramine, Pertofran
Specifics: In one case report, a mother taking 200 mg of desipramine at
bedtime had milk/plasma ratios of 0.4 to 0.9 with milk levels ranging between
17-35 µg/L.

T½= 7-60 hours   Oral= 90%   Peak= 4-6 hours
LRC= L2

DOTHIEPIN   AAP: May be of concern

Trade: Prothiaden
Can/Aus/UK:
Specifics: Dothiepin appears in breastmilk in a concentration of 11 µg/L
following a dose of 75 mg/day, while the maternal plasma level was 33 µg/L.
If the infant ingests 150 mL/kg/day of milk, the total daily dose of dothiepin
ingested by the infant in this case would be approximately 1.65 µg/kg/day,
approximately 1/650th of the adult dose.

T½= 14.4-23.9 hours   Oral= 30%   Peak= 3 hours
LRC= L2

CITALOPRAM   AAP: Not Reviewed

Trade: Celexa
Can/Aus/UK:
Specifics: The newest SSRI, citalopram enters milk in low levels. Estimated
daily intake for an infant would be approximately 4.3 µg/kg/day. This would
be less than 5.9% of the weight-adjusted maternal dose. No untoward effects
were reported in breastfed infants.

T½= 36 hours   Oral= 80%   Peak= 2-4 hours
LRC= L3

FLUOXETINE   AAP: May be of concern

Trade: Prozac, Sarafem
Can/Aus/UK: Prozac, Apo-Fluoxetine, Novo-Fluoxetine, Lovan, Zactin
Specifics: Fluoxetine and its metabolite norfluoxetine have very long half-
lives. Several reports indicate high plasma levels in some infants. Symptoms
reported include colic, insomnia, tremors, crying, hyperthermia. Use during
pregnancy, followed by use during lactation may be inadvisable. Use
cautiously in premature or newborns infants. Its use in older infants (> 2-4

months) is less risky.
T½= 2-3 days(fluoxetine)   Oral= 100%   Peak= 1.5 - 12 hours
LRC= L2 in older infants
        L3 if used in neonatal period

FLUVOXAMINE   AAP: Not Reviewed

Trade: Luvox
Can/Aus/UK: Luvox, Apo-Fluvoxamine, Alti-Fluvoxamine, Luvox, Faverin,
Floxyfral, Myroxim
Specifics: In a case report of one 23 year old mother and following a dose
of 100 mg twice daily for 2 weeks, the maternal plasma level of fluvoxamine
base was 0.31 mg/Liter and the milk concentration was 0.09 mg/Liter. The
authors reported a theoretical dose to infant of 0.0104 mg/kg/day of
fluvoxamine, which is only 0.5% of the maternal dose.
T½= 15.6 hours   Oral= 53%   Peak= 3-8 hours
LRC= L2

CARBAMAZEPINE   AAP: Compatible

Trade: Tegretol, Epitol
Can/Aus/UK: Apo-Carbamazepine, Mazepine, Teril, Tegretol
Specifics: Monitor thyroid function and recommend CBC occasionally.
T½= 18-54 hours   Oral= 100%   Peak= 4-5 hours
LRC= L2

CLONAZEPAM   AAP: Not Reviewed

Trade: Klonopin
Can/Aus/UK: Rivotril, Apo-Clonazepam, PMS-Clonazepam, Paxam
Specifics: Reported milk levels are low, 11-13 µg/L of milk.
T½= 18-50 hours   Oral= Complete   Peak= 1-4 hours
LRC= L3

HALOPERIDOL   AAP: May be of concern

Trade: Haldol
Can/Aus/UK: Apo-Haloperidol, Haldol, Novo-Peridol, Peridol, Serenace
Specifics: Milk levels are quite low even after several weeks of therapy.
T½= 12-38 hours   Oral= 60%   Peak= 2-6 hours
LRC= L2

LITHIUM CARBONATE   AAP: May be of concern

Trade: Lithobid, Eskalith
Can/Aus/UK: Carbolith, Duralith, Lithane, Lithicarb, Camcolit, Liskonum, Phasal
Specifics: Expect lithium levels in infant to be approximately 30-40% of maternal levels. Monitor both mother and infant levels periodically. Consider valproic acid as alternative.
T½= 17-24 hours   Oral= Complete   Peak= 2-4 hours
LRC= L4

PAROXETINE   AAP: Not Reviewed

Trade: Paxil
Can/Aus/UK: Paxil, Aropax 20, Seroxat
Specifics : In a recent study of 16 mothers by Stowe,   paroxetine levels in milk were low and varied according to maternal dose.   Milk/plasma ratios varied from 0.056 to 1.3.   Milk levels ranged from approximately 17 µg/L, 45 µg/L, 70 µg/L, 92 µg/L, and 101 µg/L in mothers receiving a dose of 10, 20, 30, 40, and 50 mg/day respecti ely.   Levels of paroxetine were below the limit of detection (< 2 ng/mL) in all 16 infants.   Numerous other studies generally conclude that paroxetine can be considered relatively safe for breastfeeding infants as the absolute dose transferred is quite low.   Plasma levels in the infant were generally undetectable. Recent data suggests that a neonatal withdrawal syndrome may occur in newborns exposed in utero to paroxetine.
T½= 21 hours   Oral= Complete   Peak= 5-8 hours
LRC= L2

SERTRALINE   AAP: Not Reviewed

Trade: Zoloft
Can/Aus/UK: Zoloft, Lustral
Specifics: At this time, more than 60 breastfeeding infants have been studied following maternal use of sertraline. Thus far, no untoward effects have been reported, and in almost all cases, none was detectable in the plasma compartment of the infant. No active metabolite.
T½= 26-65 hours   Oral= Complete   Peak= 7-8 hours
LRC= L2

VALPROIC ACID   AAP: Compatible

Trade: Depakene, Depakote
Can/Aus/UK: Depakene, Novo-Valproic, Deproic, Epilim, Valpro, Convulex, Epilim

Specifics: Although an anticonvulsant, valproic acid is gaining favor as a first line treatment for mania because it has a broader index of safety than lithium. Monitor liver function.

T½= 14 hours   Oral= Complete   Peak= 1-4 hours
LRC= L2

VERAPAMIL   AAP: Compatible

Trade: Calan, Isoptin, Covera-HS
Can/Aus/UK: Apo-Verap, Isoptin, Novo-Veramil, Anpec, Cordilox, Veracaps SR, Berkatens, Cordilox, Univer
Specifics: Verapamil levels in milk are generally quite low, and side effects have not been noted in breastfeeding infants. Verapamil may also be used in panic and manic attacks. But because it reduces uterine contractility, discontinue prior to delivery.

T½= 3-7 hours   Oral= 90%   Peak= 1-2.2
LRC= L2

Clinical Tips:
Acute Mania:
For acute manic episodes, haloperidol and clonazepam can be briefly used without apparent sedation of the infant. Studies with breastfeeding mothers show milk levels with both of these drugs are moderate to low, with minimal effect on the infant. In patients with acute agitation or restlessness, the benzodiazepines lorazepam or clonazepam can provide temporary relief. Both can be used in breastfeeding mothers on an acute basis. Chronic use should be avoided. Sedating antidepressants such as trazodone should generally be avoided in bipolar disorder because of cycle acceleration.

Lithium, valproate, and carbamazepine have well-documented efficacy in acute mania, although the data suggests that carbamazepine, while better than placebo, may in many cases be less effective than lithium for chronic control of mania. Valproate is apparently quite effective but is best for patients with mixed mania, concurrent drug abuse, rapid cycling, and secondary mania. Doses and clinical plasma levels are virtually identical to those used in seizure disorders and laboratory monitoring for liver function and plasma levels is recommended. Transient hair loss and cognitive dulling may sometimes occur at higher doses of valproate. Increased appetite and weight gain are common side effects. Carbamazepine and valproate have been studied in breastfeeding mothers and are consider relatively safe for use in these mothers. However, the concomitant use of valproate and carbamazepine may increase the hepatotoxic metabolites of valproate.

Lithium is more effective for elated mania and less effective for mixed manic features. However, dropout rate due to side effects (GI irritation, metallic taste, tremor, cognitive dulling) in lithium-treated patients is higher than those in valproate-treated groups. Lithium transfer into milk is low to moderate. Levels attained in the infant's plasma are generally about 30-40% of the maternal levels. If mothers are accurately maintained at around 0.6 – 1.0 meq/L, then one study (and several unpublished reports) suggests the infant's levels will be around 0.3 meq/L or 10-50% of the maternal level. The infant in one study showed no untoward effects although several other reports have suggested side effects in infants, although these may have been related to the transfer of lithium in utero. Lithium is known to inhibit thyroid function, thus occasional thyroid studies in the infant are suggested. Due to numerous drug-lithium interactions, be cautious of medicating the infant as drug interactions could occur. Any change in hydration status of the infant could induce severe toxicity and should be closely monitored. If lithium is used in women who breastfeed, the infant will be exposed and should have routine monitoring of the indices affected by the particular medication. The frequency of monitoring depends on the age of the infant. A reasonable approach is monthly for 2-3 months after any increase in maternal daily dose or if side effects are observed in the infant. The available data indicates that the use of valproic acid during lactation is probably preferable to both carbamazepine and lithium. While the onset of activity of lithium is delayed (3-4 weeks), valproate acts within days.

Acute Depression:
Experimental data concerning the treatment of bipolar depression is lacking. The response rate to treatment with tricyclic antidepressants such as imipramine appears good. Trials comparing the SSRIs such as fluoxetine and paroxetine with imipramine do not show the SSRIs more effective, but the side effect profile was significantly less with the SSRIs. Bupropion has also been found quite effective and consensus groups suggest that it and the SSRIs may be preferred agents in the treatment of depression in patients with bipolar disease. The tricyclic antidepressants have fallen into disfavor due to the likelihood of sedation, weight gain, anticholinergic effects, and acute toxicity. Because of the long half-life of fluoxetine, other SSRIs are probably preferred and include sertraline and paroxetine. Current studies also clearly suggest that prolonged use of antidepressants may significantly increase the risk of severe manic or hypomanic episodes and destabilize the course of illness. Hence, the use of antidepressants is presently only recommended during the depressive episodes. Thus the shorter half-life SSRIs are probably preferred over fluoxetine. Fluoxetine, paroxetine and sertraline have been well studied and found reasonably safe in breastfeeding patients. Data on paroxetine and sertraline show minimal transfer of these agents to breastfed infants. Fluoxetine transfer into milk and subsequent infant levels are higher although they are well tolerated in older infants. Bupropion levels in milk are considered low and non-clinical although it should not be used in patients subject to convulsive seizures. This would probably include mothers whose infants have seizure disorders or those subject to febrile seizures.

Maintenance Treatment:
Bipolar disorder is in most instances recurrent and chronic, with almost no tendency to mature out of the disorder. However, the long-term studies of lithium as maintenance therapy have been disappointing. In fact, some studies have found the outcome was no better on chronic lithium therapy than no therapy. While partially due to inadequate plasma levels, patient compliance with lithium is poor due to problems such as weight gain, hypothyroidism, polydipsia, acne, and polyuria. Recent studies have suggested that divalproex is just as effective if not better than lithium and is generally better tolerated than lithium. With chronic use, divalproex has its problems such as transient hair loss (selenium and zinc may help), weight gain and increased appetite, and cognitive dulling(dose related).

Suggested Reading:

1.   Llewellyn A, Stowe ZN, Strader JR. The use of lithium and management of women with bipolar disorder during pregnancy and lactation. J. Clin. Psychiatry 1998 59(suppl 6):57-64.
2.   Potter WZ. Bipolar depression: specific treatments. J Clin Psychiatry. 1998;59 Suppl 18:30-6. Review.
3.   Goodwin FK, et al. Understanding manic-depressive illness. Arch Gen Psychiatry. 1998 Jan;55(1):23-5. Review.
4.   Leibenluft E. Issues in the treatment of women with bipolar illness. J Clin Psychiatry. 1997;58 Suppl 15:5-11. Review.
5.   Post RM, et al. Algorithms for bipolar mania. Mod Probl Pharmacopsychiatry. 1997;25:114-45. Review.
6.   Bowden CL. In: Treatment of bipolar disorder. In Schatzberg AF, Nemeroff CB, editors: Essentials of Clinical Psychopharmacology. Washington DC, 2001. American Psychiatric Publishing, Inc.

Cardiac Arrhythmias

Principles of Therapy:
Arrhythmias are primarily rapid or abnormal changes in rhythm of the heart. Symptoms include a pounding heart (palpitations), fatigue, dyspnea, syncope, angina, heart failure. The medications used vary from the beta-blockers, calcium channel blockers, to special antiarrhythmic agents. For the purposes of this section, all of the medications used for arrhythmias are included, but the list is shorted due to limited research in breastfeeding patients. Because arrhythmias present in a host of different patterns, certain medications are only used for certain arrhythmias and the reader is cautioned that many of the included medications are not interchangeable.

ADENOSINE   **AAP:** Not Reviewed

    Trade: Adenocard
    Can/Aus/UK:
    Specifics: Adenosine is a Class IV antiarrhythmic agent. Its half-life is brief, less than 10 seconds. It would not be orally bioavailable nor likely to ever enter milk.
    T½= < 10 seconds   Oral= 0%   Peak= instant
    LRC= L3

ATENOLOL   **AAP:** Compatible

    Trade: Tenoretic, Tenormin
    Can/Aus/UK: Apo-Atenolol, Tenormin, Anselol, Noten, Tenlol, Tensig, Antipress
    Specifics: Atenolol is a second line choice beta-blocker, although it has been used in many breastfeeding women. Metoprolol or propranolol should be considered first line.
    T½= 6.1 hours   Oral= 50-60%   Peak= 2-4 hours
    LRC= L3

DIGOXIN   **AAP:** Compatible

    Trade: Lanoxin, Lanoxicaps
    Can/Aus/UK: Lanoxin, Novo-Digoxin
    Specifics: Only minimal amounts transferred into milk. Effect on infant is subclinical.
    T½= 39 hours   Oral= 65-85%   Peak= 1.5-3 hours
    LRC= L2

DISOPYRAMIDE   **AAP:** Compatible

Trade: Norpace, Napamide
Can/Aus/UK: Norpace, Rythmodan, Isomide
Specifics: Small amounts in milk. No plasma levels noted in infants.
T½= 8.3-11.65 hours   Oral= 60-83%   Peak= 2.3 hours
LRC= L2

ESMOLOL   **AAP:** Not Reviewed

Trade: Brevibloc
Can/Aus/UK: Brevibloc
Specifics: Although no breastfeeding data are available, esmolol is the same class as propranolol and has a very short half-life.
T½= 9 minutes   Oral= Poor   Peak= 15 min.
LRC= L3

FLECAINIDE   **AAP:** Approved

Trade: Tambocor
Can/Aus/UK: Tambocor
Specifics: Flecainide is a potent antiarrhythmic. In a study of 11 patients receiving 100 mg oral flecainide, average milk levels ranged from 270-1529 µg/L (mean= 953 µg/L). Assuming the highest, the average daily intake via milk in an infant would be 1.07 mg. In a normal 4 kg infant, the average plasma concentration in a breastfed infant would not be expected to exceed about 62 ng/mL. The average plasma level in infants treated with therapeutic doses is 360 ng/mL.
T½= 7-22 hours   Oral= 90%   Peak= 4.5 hours
LRC= L4

LIDOCAINE   **AAP:** Compatible

Trade: Xylocaine
Can/Aus/UK: Xylocard, Xylocaine, Lignocaine, EMLA
Specifics: Lidocaine levels in milk are extremely low, even following high maternal IV doses.
T½= 1.8 hours   Oral= <35%   Peak=Immediate
LRC= L3

METOPROLOL   **AAP:** Compatible

Trade: Toprol XL, Lopressor
Can/Aus/UK: Apo-Metoprolol, Betaloc, Lopressor, Novo-Metoprol, Minax
Specifics: First line choice of beta-blocker for breastfeeding women. Milk

levels are minimal. Side effects in infant are minimal.

T½= 3-7 hours   Oral= 40-50%   Peak= 2.5-3 hours
LRC= L3

MEXILETINE HCL   AAP: Compatible

Trade: Mexitil
Can/Aus/UK: Mexitil, Novo-Mexiletine
Specifics: Reported milk levels are extremely small. No side effects were noted.

T½= 9.2 hours   Oral= 90%   Peak= 2-3 hours
LRC= L2

PHENYTOIN   AAP: Compatible

Trade: Dilantin
Can/Aus/UK: Dilantin, Novo-Phenytoin, Epanutin
Specifics: Amount transferred in milk is minimal. Infant plasma levels are low to undetectable.

T½= 6-24 hours   Oral= 70-100%   Peak= 4-12 hours
LRC= L2

PROCAINAMIDE   AAP: Compatible

Trade: Pronestyl, Procan
Can/Aus/UK: Pronestyl, Procan SR, Apo-Procainamide
Specifics: Levels in milk are modest to low. No untoward effects have been reported.

T½= 3.0 hours   Oral= 75-90%   Peak= 0.75-2.5 hours
LRC= L3

PROPRANOLOL   AAP: Compatible

Trade: Inderal
Can/Aus/UK: Detensol, Inderal, Novo-Pranol, Deralin, Cardinol
Specifics: Propranolol is an ideal beta-blocker for breastfeeding women. Numerous studies show minimal milk levels and minimal to no side effects in the infant.

T½= 3-5 hours   Oral= 30%   Peak= 60-90 min.
LRC= L3

PROPAFENONE   **AAP:** Compatible

Trade: Rythmol
Can/Aus/UK: Arythmol
Specifics: Propafenone is a class 1C antiarrhythmic agent with structural similarities to propranolol. In a mother receiving 300 mg three times daily, maternal serum levels of propafenone and 5-OH-propafenone(active metabolite) were 219 µg/L and 86 µg/L respectively. The breastmilk level of parafenone and 5-OH-propafenone was 32 µg/L and 47 µg/L respectively. The authors estimate that the daily intake of drug and active metabolite in their infant (3.3 kg) would have been 16 µg and 24 µg per day respectively.
T½= 2-10 hours   Oral= 12%   Peak= 2-3 hours
LRC= L2

QUINIDINE   **AAP:** Compatible

Trade: Quinaglute, Quinidex
Can/Aus/UK: Apo-Quinidine, Cardioquin, Novo-Quinidin, Kinidin Durules, Kiditard
Specifics: Milk levels are quite low (<1% of dose). Because quinidine is stored in the liver, occasional liver enzyme studies in infant may be advisable after long-term exposure.
T½= 6-8 hours   Oral= 80%   Peak= 1-2 hours
LRC= L2

SOTALOL   **AAP:** Compatible

Trade: Betapace
Can/Aus/UK: Sotacor, Apo-Sotalol, Rylosol, Cardol
Specifics: Although milk levels appear high, no evidence of absorption in infants was noted, nor any side effects. Least preferred of this group.
T½= 12 hours   Oral= 90-100%   Peak= 2.5 - 4 hours
LRC= L3

VERAPAMIL   **AAP:** Compatible

Trade: Calan, Isoptin, Covera-HS
Can/Aus/UK: Apo-Verap, Isoptin, Novo-Veramil, Anpec, Cordilox, Veracaps SR, Berkatens, Univer
Specifics: Verapamil levels in milk are generally quite low, and side effects have not been noted in breastfeeding infants. Verapamil may also be used in panic and manic attacks. But because it reduces uterine contractility, discontinue prior to delivery.
T½= 3-7 hours   Oral= 90%   Peak= 1-2.2 hours
LRC= L2

WARFARIN

AAP: Compatible

Trade: Coumadin, Panwarfin
Can/Aus/UK: Coumadin, Warfilone, Marevan
Specifics: Warfarin is highly protein bound. Milk levels are virtually undetectable. In numerous studies, no effects on breastfeeding infants have been reported.

$T\frac{1}{2}$= 1-2.5 days   Oral= Complete   Peak= 0.5-3 days
LRC= L2

Clinical Tips:

The choice of an antiarrhythmic is largely dependent on the type of arrhythmia. Of the numerous newer antiarrhythmic drugs, few have been studied in breastfeeding mothers. Of the beta-blockers, propranolol and metoprolol are preferred. While atenolol has been commonly used, and is approved by the AAP, one case of neonatal bradycardia has been reported. No reports on esmolol have been found, but it is structurally similarly to propranolol, and its short half-life suggest that its milk levels may be low. Lidocaine has been studied in several breastfeeding mothers, some at high doses (965 mg over 7 hours). The maximum dose via milk is likely less than 120 µg/kg/day. In four studies thus far, all the authors suggest it is safe to breastfeed following lidocaine therapy.

Studies on flecainide and propafenone indicate low milk levels and the authors suggest that no untoward effects were noted. Reported milk levels of verapamil vary but none has yet been detected in the infant's plasma compartment. Due to high milk levels and untoward effects, do not use amiodarone in breastfeeding mothers.

Suggested Reading:

1. Arrhythmias. Curr Opin Cardiol. 1997 Jan;12(1):B1-25.
2. Amar D. Cardiac arrhythmias. Chest Surg Clin N Am. 1998 Aug;8(3):479-93, vii. Review.

Congestive Heart Failure

Principles of Therapy:

Chronic congestive heart failure results from various etiologies including valvular heart disease, hypertension, ischemic heart disease, peri-partum cardiomyopathy, and primarily myocardial diseases. Presenting symptoms include dyspnea, fatigue, edema, pulmonary venous hypertension, and decreased cardiac output. The classic enlargement of the heart is pathognomic of impending pump failure. Therapeutic options include: diuretics, digitalis, beta-blockers (rarely), calcium channel blockers, nitrate vasodilators, antiarrhythmic drugs, and other antihypertensives. The objective of pharmacotherapy is to improve cardiac output, reduce fluid overload, reduce hypertension, reduce peripheral resistance, and increase exercise tolerance.

ATENOLOL   **AAP:** Approved

Trade:
Can/Aus/UK:
Specifics: Data published thus far suggests milk levels are highly variable but seem higher than others in this family.   Milk levels vary from approximately 0.66 mg/L (25 mg maternal dose) to 1.7 mg/L (100 mg maternal dose).   While one case of severe hypotension has been reported, this is probably rare with most normal doses. Some caution is recommended.
T½= 6.1 hours   Oral= 50%   Peak= 2-4 hours
LRC= L3

BENAZEPRIL HCL   **AAP:** Not Reviewed

Trade: Lotensin
Can/Aus/UK:
Specifics: May be suitable, but studies are incomplete. Benazepril is poorly bioavailability. Captopril may be a preferred ACE inhibitor.
T½= 10-11 hours   Oral= 37%   Peak= 0.5 - 1 hr.
LRC= L3
        L4 if used in neonatal period

CAPTOPRIL   **AAP:** Compatible

Trade: Capoten
Can/Aus/UK: Capoten, Apo-Capto, Novo-Captopril, Acenorm, Enzace, Acepril
Specifics: Milk levels are very low (4.7 µg/L of milk). No adverse effect in 12 infants studied. Avoid in early neonatal periods because infants may be excessively sensitive.

70

T½= 2.2 hours   Oral= 60-75%   Peak= 1 hr.
LRC= L3 if used after 30 days
          L4 if used early postpartum

DIGOXIN   AAP: Compatible

Trade: Lanoxin, Lanoxicaps
Can/Aus/UK: Lanoxin, Novo-Digoxin
Specifics: Only minimal amounts transferred into milk. Effect on infant is subclinical.
T½= 39 hours   Oral= 65-85%   Peak= 1.5-3 hours
LRC= L2

DOPAMINE-DOBUTAMINE   AAP: Not Reviewed

Trade: Intropin
Can/Aus/UK:
Specifics: Not orally bioavailable to the infant.
T½= 2 minutes   Oral= Poor   Peak= 5 minutes.
LRC= L2

ENALAPRIL MALEATE   AAP: Compatible

Trade: Vasotec
Can/Aus/UK: Vasotec, Amprace, Renitec, Innovace
Specifics: Studies show levels are quite low, but they were not done at steady state. Captopril or benazepril may be preferred. Avoid in early neonatal periods, infants may be excessively sensitive.
T½= 35 hours(metabolite)   Oral= 60%   Peak= 0.5-1.5 hours
LRC= L2
          L4 if used early postpartum

FUROSEMIDE   AAP: Not Reviewed

Trade: Lasix
Can/Aus/UK: Apo-Furosemide, Novo-Semide, Lasix, Frusemide, Uremide, Frusid
Specifics: Furosemide levels in milk are unreported but are believed to be low. Oral bioavailability of furosemide in neonates is extremely poor.
T½= 92 minutes   Oral= 60-70%   Peak= 1-2 hours
LRC= L3

HYDRALAZINE   **AAP:** Compatible

Trade: Apresoline
Can/Aus/UK: Apresoline, Novo-Hylazin, Apo-Hydralazine, Alphapress,
Apresoline
Specifics: Milk levels are small and the amount ingested by infant is
generally subclinical.   Good choice for pre-eclampsia, gestational, and
postpartum hypertension.
T½= 1.5-8 hours   Oral= 30-50%   Peak= 2 hours
LRC= L2

METOPROLOL   **AAP:** Compatible

Trade: Toprol XL, Lopressor
Can/Aus/UK: Apo-Metoprolol, Betaloc, Lopressor, Novo-Metoprol, Minax
Specifics: First line choice of beta-blocker for breastfeeding women. Milk
levels are minimal. Side effects in infant are minimal.
T½= 3-7 hours   Oral= 40-50%   Peak= 2.5-3 hours
LRC= L3

NIFEDIPINE   **AAP:** Compatible

Trade: Adalat, Procardia
Can/Aus/UK: Adalat, Apo-Nifed, Novo-Nifedin, Nu-Nifed, Nifecard,
Nyefax, Nefensar XL
Specifics: Milk levels of this calcium channel blocker are quite low. Its use
in angina and CHF is not preferred.
T½= 1.8-7 hours   Oral= 50%   Peak= 45 min-4 hours
LRC= L2

NITRENDIPINE   **AAP:** Not Reviewed

Trade: Baypress
Can/Aus/UK:
Specifics: Estimated intake per day would be 1.7 µg (0.95% of maternal
dose).
T½= 8-11 hours   Oral= 16-20%   Peak= 1-2 hours
LRC= L2

VERAPAMIL   **AAP:** Compatible

Trade: Calan, Isoptin, Covera-HS
Can/Aus/UK: Apo-Verap, Isoptin, Novo-Veramil, Anpec, Cordilox,
Veracaps SR, Berkatens, Cordilox, Univer
Specifics: Verapamil levels in milk are generally quite low, and side effects

have not been noted in breastfeeding infants. Verapamil may also be used in panic and manic attacks. But because it reduces uterine contractility, discontinue prior to delivery. Use of CCBs in CHF is not generally recommended at present.

T½= 3-7 hours   Oral= 90%   Peak= 1-2.2
LRC= L2

NIMODIPINE   AAP: Not Reviewed

Trade: Nimotop
Can/Aus/UK: Nimotop
Specifics: Breastmilk levels are reported to be very low in at least several studies. No untoward effects were noted in the infants.

T½= 9 hours   Oral= 13%   Peak= 1 hour
LRC= L2

SPIRONOLACTONE   AAP: Approved

Trade: Aldactone
Can/Aus/UK: Aldactone, Novospiroton, Spiractin
Specifics: Spironolactone is metabolized to canrenone, which is known to be secreted into breastmilk. In one mother receiving 25 mg of spironolactone, at 2 hours the maternal serum and milk concentrations of canrenone were 144 and 104 µg/L respectively. At 14.5 hours, the corresponding values for serum and milk were 92 and 47 µg/L respectively. The estimated dose an infant would ingest was 0.2% of maternal dose/day. Use cautiously, if at all, with ACE inhibitors.

T½= 10-35 hours   Oral= 70%   Peak= 1-2 hours
LRC= L2

Clinical Tips:

Treatment of early stage heart failure offers the best chance at long-term survival. At this time, loop diuretics and ACE inhibitors have the best record. The combination of spironolactone along with an ACE inhibitor may provide some added benefit as recent studies suggest significant benefit of a potassium-sparing diuretic in congestive heart failure (CHF) patients. Of the loop diuretics, furosemide is generally recommended in breastfeeding patients rather than bumetanide because it is poorly bioavailable in the infant. Bumetanide is not absolutely contraindicated in breastfeeding mothers, rather we have no breastmilk data on this product as of yet. ACE inhibitors, particularly captopril, have been found to greatly reduce morbidity in these patients and experts agree that 50-75% of CHF patients should receive ACE inhibitors. Although other ACE inhibitors are probably fine, captopril is ideal due to its low milk levels and studies showing it significantly reduces morbidity in patients with congestive heart failure. Again, caution is urged in neonates as they have poor control of their blood pressure and cases of hypotension have been reported in mothers ingesting ACE inhibitors prior to delivery. After several weeks postpartum and in full term, stable infants, the use of ACE inhibitors in breastfeeding mothers is less hazardous. As of yet, the only potassium-sparing diuretic studied in breastfeeding mothers has been spironolactone. Only 0.2% of the maternal dose transfers to the infant and its use is approved by the AAP. At present we do not have data on amiloride or triamterene. The use of ACE inhibitors with potassium-sparing diuretics is somewhat risky, as elevated serum potassium levels may result. Potassium-sparing diuretics should probably be used cautiously or not at all in patients taking ACE inhibitors.

The use of calcium channel blockers (CCB) in CHF is controversial and in general are not recommended as they tend to worsen the syndrome. These include nifedipine, diltiazem, and verapamil. Newer CCBs such as amlodipine (Norvasc) may reduce death rate in some subgroups, but the effect seems minimal. No data on its use in breastfeeding mothers are available.

Previously, the use of beta-blockers in CHF was discouraged as they were believed to reduce the pumping action of the heart (ionotropy). New data seems to suggest that certain beta-blockers may have significant benefits to heart failure patients. Some of the beta-blockers now recommended include atenolol, carvedilol (Coreg), metoprolol (Lopressor), bisoprolol (Zebeta). Of this family, atenolol has been associated with hypotension in breastfed infants, but this may be rare. Many patients have breastfed using this beta-blocker without problems, but some caution is recommended. At present metoprolol is the only beta-blocker which is known to pass poorly to breastfed infants, to have minimal side effects in breastfed infants, and to be rated usually compatible by the AAP. At present we do not have breastfeeding data on carvedilol or bisoprolol. However, the use of beta-blockers in CHF patients must be approached cautiously because beta-blockers reduce pumping action and worsening of heart failure may occur. Fatigue, lethargy, exacerbation of asthma, sexual dysfunction, and other side effects are common with their use. In breastfed infants, severe hypotension has been reported (although rarely) in patients consuming atenolol and acebutolol so caution is recommended with these two agents.

Digoxin, although only moderately efficacious, is still the recommended inotropic agent of choice. Hydralazine can be used, but it is often poorly efficacious. Dopamine and dobutamine are not orally bioavailable to the infant and can be used if needed. For other antiarrhythmic agents, see 'Cardiac Antiarrhythmias'.

Suggested Reading:

1.   Guthery D, et al. Congestive heart failure. J Am Acad Nurse Pract. 1998 Jan;10(1):31-8; quiz 39-41. Review.
2.   Cohn JN. The management of chronic heart failure. N Engl J Med. 1996 Aug 15;

335(7):490-8. Review.

3.   Keogh A. Heart failure--outlooks and strategies for treatment. Aust N Z J Med. 1997 Aug;27(4):485-91. Review.

4.   Cohn JN. Overview of the treatment of heart failure. Am J Cardiol. 1997 Dec 4;80(11A):2L-6L. Review.

5.   Ahmed O. Management of congestive heart failure in primary care settings. Compr Ther. 1997 Jul;23(7):472-6. Review.

6.   Fletcher L, Thomas D. Congestive heart failure: understanding the pathophysiology and management. J Am Acad Nurse Pract. 2001 ; 13(6):249-57.

7.   Rich MW. Management of heart failure in the elderly. Heart Fail Rev. 2002 Jan;7(1):89-97.

8.   Hanes DS, Weir MR. The beta-blockers: are they as protective in hypertension as in other cardiovascular conditions? J Clin Hypertens (Greenwich). 2001 Jul-Aug;3(4):236-43.

9.   Ferdinand KC. Update in pharmacologic treatment of hypertension. Cardiol Clin. 2001 May;19(2):279-94, v.

Conjunctivitis, Bacterial

Principles of Therapy:
Conjunctivitis is the most common eye disorder and may be acute or chronic. Acute bacterial conjunctivitis is characterized by an abrupt onset of conjunctival hyperemia (redness), mucopurulent discharge, and a foreign body sensation. Most cases are due to bacterial or viral infections, although some are due to allergy or chemical irritants. In bacterial conjunctivitis, the most common organisms are staphylococci, streptococci, haemophilus, pseudomonas, and Moraxella. However, chlamydia and gonococcus are also prevalent. All may produce a mucopurulent discharge although changes in visual acuity is uncommon.

AZITHROMYCIN   **AAP:** Not Reviewed

Trade: Zithromax
Can/Aus/UK: Zithromax
Specifics: Azithromycin levels in milk are very low. In one study of a patient who received 1 gm initially, followed by two 500mg doses at 24 hr intervals, the concentration of azithromycin in breastmilk varied from 0.64 mg/L (initially) to 2.8 mg/L on day 3.
T1/2= 48-68 hours   Oral= 37%   Peak= 3-4 hours
LRC= L2

CEFTRIAXONE   **AAP**: Not Reviewed
Trade: Rocephin
Can/Aus/UK: Rocephin
Specifics: Small amounts are transferred into milk (3-4% of maternal serum level). Following a 1 gm IM dose, breastmilk levels were approximately 0.5-0.7 mg/L at between 4-8 hours. The estimated mean milk levels at steady state were 3-4 mg/L. Another source indicates that following a 2 g/d dose and at steady state, approximately 4.4 % of dose penetrates into milk. In this study, the maximum breastmilk concentration was 7.89 mg/L after prolonged therapy (7days). Using this data, the weight-adjusted relative infant dose would only be 0.35% of the maternal dose. Poor oral absorption of ceftriaxone would further limit systemic absorption by the infant.
T½= 7.3 hours   Oral= Poor   Peak= 1 hour
LRC= L2

CIPROFLOXACIN   AAP: Compatible

Trade: Cipro, Ciloxan
Can/Aus/UK: Cipro, Ciloxan, Ciproxin
Specifics: Ophthalmic use of ciprofloxacin produces minimal plasma levels and the amount entering milk would be minimal.
T½= 4.1 hours   Oral= 50-85%   Peak= 0.5-2.3 hours
LRC= L4

ERYTHROMYCIN   AAP: Compatible

Trade: E-mycin, Ery-tab, Eryc, Ilosone
Can/Aus/UK: E-mycin, Eryc, Erythromid, Novo-Rythro, PCE,Ilotyc, EMU-V, Ilosone, EES, Erythrocin, Ceplac, Erycen
Specifics: Reported milk levels are less than 1.5 mg/Liter, generally considered subclinical.
T½= 1.5-2 hours   Oral= Variable   Peak= 2-4 hours
LRC= L1

OFLOXACIN   AAP: Not Reviewed

Trade: Floxin
Can/Aus/UK: Floxin, Ocuflox, Tarivid
Specifics: In one study in lactating women who received 400 mg oral doses twice daily, drug concentrations in breastmilk averaged 0.05-2.41 mg/L in milk (24 hours and 2 hours post-dose respectively). Milk levels are much lower than ciprofloxacin levels.
T½= 5-7 hours   Oral= 98 %   Peak= 0.5-2 hours
LRC= L3

TETRACYCLINE   AAP: Compatible

Trade: Achromycin, Sumycin, Terramycin
Can/Aus/UK: Achromycin, Aureomycin, Tetracyn, Mysteclin, Tetrex, Tetrachel
Specifics: Milk levels are low, and oral bioavailability in milk is low. In a study of 5 lactating women receiving 500 mg PO four times daily, the breastmilk concentrations ranged from 0.43 mg/L to 2.58 mg/L. Levels in infants were below the limit of detection. Chronic use over months may not be advisable due to dental staining.
T½= 6-12 hours   Oral= 75%   Peak= 1.5-4 hours
LRC= L2
       L4 if used chronically

Clinical Tips:

Hyperacute bacterial conjunctivitis is a severe, sight-threatening infection that warrants immediate care. It is characterized by copious yellow-green purulent discharge of abrupt onset. Symptoms also include redness, irritation, tenderness, lid swelling, and conjunctival chemosis(edema). The most frequent causes of hyperacute bacterial conjunctivitis are *N. gonorrhoeae* and *Neisseria meningitidis*. Gonococcal infections occur most commonly in newborns (5 days postpartum) and young adults(sexually active). All patients should be treated with systemic antibiotics supplemented by topical ocular antibiotics and saline. The systemic agent of choice is ceftriaxone (Rocephin) due to prevalence of resistance of *N. gonorrhoeae* although a two-week course of systemic erythromycin is effective for Gonococcal infections.

Acute bacterial conjunctivitis typically presents with irritation, burning, excessive tearing, and usually a mucopurulent discharge. Eye matting on awakening, conjunctival swelling, and mild eyelid edema may be noted. The most common pathogens are *S. pneumoniae, H. influenzae,* and *Staphlococcus aureus*. Topical preparations suitable for these milder infections include erythromycin ointment, bacitracin-polymyxin B ointment, or trimethoprim-polymyxin B (Polytrim). While the aminoglycosides can be used in some cases, they do not cover gram -positive species as well, including staphlococcus and streptococcus.

For chlamydial keratoconjunctivitis, oral erythromycin, azithromycin, or tetracycline are suitable. Most recently, the fluoroquinolones which include ciprofloxacin (Ciloxan) , ofloxacin(Ocuflox), and norfloxacin (Chibroxin) are becoming more popular and are very effective particularly in those patients hypersensitive to erythromycins or penicillins. Although they are not cleared for pediatric use, the amount of absorption following ocular administration is minimal. Further, their cost is somewhat prohibitive. These agents should probably be reserved for resistant cases that have documented sensitivity studies showing efficacy of these agents. The ophthalmic use of chloramphenicol while effective, has been associated with subsequent cases of aplastic anemia and thus should be avoided.

Suggested Reading:

1. Morrow GL, et al. Conjunctivitis. Am Fam Physician. 1998 Feb 15;57(4):735-46. Review.
2. Friedlaender MH. A review of the causes and treatment of bacterial and allergic conjunctivitis. Clin Ther. 1995 Sep-Oct;17(5):800-10; discussion 779. Review.
3. Weber CM, et al. Acute red eye. Differentiating viral conjunctivitis from other, less common causes. Postgrad Med. 1997 May;101(5):185-6, 189-92, 195-6. Review.

Contraception

It is generally recognized that most women who breastfeed exclusively enter a period of lactational amenorrhea. During this time potential for ovulation is reduced. Conception rates during lactational amenorrhea vary over time since delivery. During the first 6 months post-partum, in the exclusively breastfeeding woman experiencing amenorrhea, the chances of conception are approximately 0.5 to 2%. For this effectiveness, supplementation should be avoided and the longest nighttime feeding interval should be no longer than six hours with 8 or greater feedings daily. Over the next 6 months chances for conception increase though some reduction in fertility is preserved while amenorrhea persists. In mothers providing exclusive breastmilk for their young infants but separated from the infants and therefore using milk expression, the effectiveness of LAM may be slightly decreased with an anticipated pregnancy rate of about 5% at 6 months. Some contraceptives when used injudiciously can seriously impact breastmilk production, and reduce the growth rate of the infant. This most often occurs with estrogens and occasionally with progestin products. For this reason, it is well known that during the first 6-8 weeks postpartum, oral contraceptives containing estrogens should be strongly discouraged. Actually most authorities agree that breastfeeding women should avoid estrogen-containing products throughout breastfeeding. Progestin-only products are generally preferred for breastfeeding mothers, as they have consistently been found to produce fewer effects on breastmilk production.

BARRIER CONTRACEPTIVES

Barrier methods of contraception such as diaphragms and condoms have no impact on milk production and though they offer reduced efficacy compared to many alternatives, they may be satisfactory during lactation due to the relative reduction in fertility afforded by lactation. Barrier methods may require the use of vaginal lubricants during lactation due to the vaginal atrophy frequently experienced by recently post-partum and lactating women. The following table suggests the efficacy expected in the "typical" user, not specific for lactating women.

Method	"Typical" User Efficacy
Spermicide	79%
Condom (Male)	88%
Diaphragm	82%
Cervical Cap	82%

MECHANICAL CONTRACEPTIVES (IUD)

Mechanical methods of contraception may or may not have hormonal effects that could be pertinent to lactation. Those which are non-hormonal do not impact milk supply. A major disadvantage to the intrauterine device or IUD is that it requires insertion and removal by a health care provider. Some older information suggests that there may be a slight increased risk of uterine perforation upon insertion of the IUD in lactating women though this risk is quite small and should not dissuade IUD use in otherwise good candidates for this contraceptive option. Currently available alternative IUD's may be the non-hormonal copper containing type or the hormonal progesterone containing type. Progesterone doses in the IUD are low and are felt to exert a local effect on the endometrial lining which minimizes vaginal bleeding. To what extent these progesterone IUD's result in blood levels which could impact lactation has not been well investigated but is speculated to be less than that of other progesterone contraceptive methods. Effectiveness of the IUD for contraception is approximately 97%.

COPPER IUD   AAP: Not Reviewed
    Trade: Copper T 380 A
    Specifics: Copper containing IUD. May be used for up to 10 years.
    Contraindicated in Wilson's   disease and copper allergy.
    LRC = L3

PROGESTIN IUD   AAP: Not Reviewed
    Trade: Progestesert, Mirena (levonorgestrel releasing)
    Specifics: Progestesert requires replacement every year. Mirena may be left
    in place for up to 5 years. Potential for hormonal effects on lactation may be
    similar to other progestin containing contraceptives. Failure rates for the
    levonorgestrel releasing IUD are <1%. See section below.
    LRC = L3

PROGESTIN CONTAINING CONTRACEPTIVES

Progestin only contraceptives are generally preferred in breastfeeding women over combination hormonal contraceptive containing estrogen. Depending on the particular contraceptive, these methods are also highly efficacious. Often progestin-only contraceptives result in irregular menstruation in non-lactating women. In lactating women, however, amenorrhea is a frequent occurrence and the woman should be counseled about this anticipated result. Progestin contraceptives can have a dose dependent impact on milk supply though the amount typically used for contraception is not commonly found to cause difficulties. The fall in progesterone that occurs after delivery is important in establishment of the mother's milk supply. Theoretically, initiating progestin contraception in the first few days after delivery could interfere with this natural process and result in poor milk supply. Little research has been done regarding the potential impact of early initiation of progestin contraception to provide scientific guidance. Information from those studies that have been done looking at early initiation of progesterone-only contraception do not document problems with poor milk supply or infant growth. It is prudent to begin these forms of contraception 4-6 weeks after delivery or later unless circumstances require earlier use. This would be unlikely if exclusive breastfeeding is anticipated. Progestin-only contraception is available as a daily pill, injectable medication, implantable device, vaginal ring (not presently available in US), and in IUD's. Injectable and implantable devices have the benefit of improved efficacy and less reliance on user compliance but are less easily reversible should concerns about milk supply develop. Theoretically, norethindrone-containing oral contraceptives may have some potential peripheral conversion to estrogen that levonorgestrel pills lack, however, no clinical difference has been noted with regard to lactation. Another potential concern has been the exposure of the nursing infant to hormones. Though progestins have been detected in breastmilk of mothers using these contraceptive methods, adverse outcomes have not been found in the nursing infant.

LEVONORGESTREL IMPLANTS   AAP: Compatible
Trade: Norplant
Can/Aus/UK: Norplant
Specifics: Levonorgestrel is a progestin used generally in repository form for contraception. Norplant consists of six levonorgestrel containing capsules. Contraceptive effects persist for 5 years. Failure rates for contraception are <1%.
LRC= L3

ETONOGESTREL IMPLANTS   AAP: Not Reviewed
Trade: Implanon
Can/Aus/UK:
Specifics: Etonogestrel is a progestin available in a single implantable rod providing contraception for 3 years. Failure rates for contraception are <1%. This is anticipated to be introduced into the marketplace in the next year.
LRC= L3

MEDROXYPROGESTERONE INJECTIONS   AAP: Compatible
Trade: Depo-Provera
Can/Aus/UK: Depo-Provera
Specifics: Progestin product used generally in repository form for contraception. Some information suggests that it may suppress breastmilk production in some patients. Administration should be avoided prior to 6-8 weeks post-partum if possible. A challenge with an oral progestin-only preparation prior to using a depository form of progersteone may be advisable. Depo-provera is functional for contraception for 3 month intervals

but may require substantially longer for effects to reverse. Failure rates for contraception are <1%

LRC= L1

L4 if used first 3 days postpartum

NORETHINDRONE   **AAP**: Not Reviewed

Trade: Aygestin, Norlutate, Micronor, Nor-Q.D.

Can/Aus/UK: Micronor, Norlutate, Norethisterone, Brevinor

Specifics: Commonly used in progestin-only birth control preparations. This is an ideal product to initiate birth control in breastfeeding mothers. Pills must be taken daily at roughly the same time. There is no "pill free" week. Efficacy in the typical user is about 97% (not specific to lactating women). If reduced milk production is noted, simply discontinue the medication.

T1/2= 4-13 hours   Oral= 60%   Peak= 1-2 hours

LRC= L1

ESTROGEN-CONTAINING COMBINATION CONTRACEPTIVES

Estrogen containing contraceptives are not recommended as an initial choice for breastfeeding women due to the known negative impact on milk supply. This effect is more pronounced with higher estrogen levels. Many commercially advertised "low dose" estrogen containing birth control pills are available with estrogen doses ranging from 20 to 35 µg of estrogen. If a breastfeeding woman chooses an estrogen containing contraceptive, theoretically the lower estrogen dose should have the least impact on milk supply. A 20 µg pill would be the best available option. The combination estrogen containing injectable is even less desirable due to the longer duration of activity. If reduced milk supply occurred, the effect would be expected to continue for the month period of expected efficacy. Many different progestins are available in combination oral contraceptives. The impact of the different progestins on lactation has not been well researched. Most research has focused only on the different estrogen amounts available in different pills. Various progestins have slightly different side effect profiles so differences in effect on lactation are possible. Drosperidone is a progestin that has recently been introduced to the US market which has a spironolactone like effect. Though this may be beneficial for the side effect profile of this oral contraceptive in general, there is a small theoretic risk that this could impact milk supply though scientific investigation has not been done.

ESTROGEN CONTAINING ORAL CONTRACEPTIVE PRODUCTS

Estrogen containing oral contraceptive pills contain varying amounts of ethinyl estradiol in addition to one of several different progestin compounds. These products have slightly different combinations and doses designed to given various different formulations slightly different side effect profiles. The impact of various different combinations on the lactating mother-baby dyad has not been well researched. Reduction in milk supply seems to at least be related to the amount of estrogen contained in the contraceptive. Therefore, theoretically the lowest estrogen dose available would be expected to be least detrimental to milk supply though some effect would still be expected. If this method is chosen, begin the lowest estrogen dose available after milk supply has been well established and counsel the patient about the potential for reduction in milk supply and discontinuation of the pills if milk volume reduction is noted.

ESTROGEN AND PROGESTERONE INJECTABLE   AAP: Not Reviewed
CONTRACEPTION
   Trade: Lunelle
   Can/Aus/UK:
Specifics: This contraceptive contains both estrogen (estradiol cypionate) and a progestin (medroxyprogesterone acetate). The potential impact on lactation would likely be similar to other combination estrogen containing contraceptives. A potential disadvantage to this particular method is that the injectible medication can not be stopped once it is given, therefore any adverse impact on milk supply will likely persist until the duration of the hormonal effect has passed. The contraceptive effect persists for approximately one month and the impact on lactation could be expected to be of similar duration. Failure rates for contraception are <1%
   LRC= L3

VAGINAL RING   AAP: Not Reviewed
   Trade: NuvaRing
   Can/Aus/UK:
Specifics: This flexible vaginal ring releases the estrogen ethinyl estradiol (15mgs daily) and the progestin etonogestrel (120mgs daily). Each vaginal ring is worn for 3 weeks during which hormone is released. The ring is then removed for a one week hormone free interval. No information is available regarding use in lactation but would likely be similar to low dose estrogen containing birth control pills.

TRANSDERMAL ESTROGEN PATCH   AAP: Not Reviewed
   Trade: OrthoEvra
   Can/Aus/UK:
Specifics: This contraceptive patch contains both estrogen and a progestin and is designed to release 150 µg of norelgestromin and 20 µg of ethinyl estradiol daily. The patch is applied once weekly for 3 consecutive weeks followed by one week patch free to allow for menstruation. Hormone levels after application of the patch provide contraceptive efficacy for 9 days. The effect of this contraceptive method on milk supply has not been well investigated, however it would be expected to be similar to low dose estrogen

containing oral contraceptive pills. This method would be reversible by removing the patch should alteration in milk supply be noted. Failure rates for contraception are similar to oral contraceptive pills at <1%.
LRC= L4

Post-Coital Contraception

Post-coital contraception is also known as the "morning after"pill or emergency contraception. For this to provide effectiveness in preventing pregnancy it should be initiated within 72 hours of unprotected intercourse. The progesterone only form described below is slightly more efficacious and is less likely to negatively impact lactation.

PROGESTIN-ONLY POST-COITAL   AAP: Not Reviewed
CONTRACEPTION
    Trade: Plan B
    Can/Aus/UK:
    Specifics: This form of emergency contraception includes 2 doses of levonorgestrel 0.75mgs taken 12 hours apart and initiated as soon as possible but within 72 hours of unprotected intercourse. The efficacy of this method is approximately 85%. This form of emergency contraception is better tolerated in terms of causing less nausea than its estrogen-containing counterpart. It would theoretically also be better in breastfeeding patients as it does not contain estrogen and would have less potential to negatively impact milk supply.
    LRC= L3

COMBINATION HORMONAL POST-COITAL   AAP: Not Reviewed
CONTRACEPTION
    Trade: Preven
    Can/Aus/UK:
    Specifics: This form of emergency contraception includes 2 doses of levonorgestrel 0.25 mgs and ethinyl estradiol 0.05 mgs taken 12 hours apart and initiated as soon as possible but within 72 hours of unprotected intercourse. The efficacy of this method is estimated to be between 55 and 75%. This form of emergency contraception may cause nausea (approximately 50%) and an anti-emetic medication is frequently prescribed along with this medication. Due to the relatively high estrogen dose (100 μg/day) this form of contraception would be anticipated to have a negative impact on milk supply. Fortunately, this high estrogen dose is only used for one day so the effect would be anticipated to be temporary.
    LRC= L4

Clinical Tips:

Estrogen-containing birth control products can seriously reduce breastmilk production and should be avoided at least for the first two months postpartum. Most authorities agree that breastfeeding women should avoid estrogen-containing products throughout breastfeeding. Estrogens significantly reduce lactose and protein production in the alveolar epithelial cells that produce milk, hence milk volume and protein content is reduced in many patients. The longer one can wait to use these products, the less the inhibitory response. The injectable estrogen containing products are likely the least desirable alternatives. These would not be easily reversible if a decrease in milk production were to occur. During the early postpartum period, progestin-only products are strongly recommended. If the patient is non-compliant then the injectable medroxyprogesterone may be used. However, there are reports suggesting that even with Depo-Provera some patients may have reduced milk supply, particularly if used prior to 6 weeks postpartum. For this reason, a preliminary trial of low-dose oral progestin-only products (norethindrone 0.35 mg, norgestrel 0.075 mg) is suggested. If the mother's milk supply is sustained following use of these products, then the repository form of medroxyprogesterone (Depo-Provera) or the implantable levonorgestrel (Norplant) system could probably be used safely. Frequently reported break through bleeding experienced by the non-lactating woman using progestin-only products is much less common in the post-partum period of breastfeeding mothers. Numerous studies show that the amount of progestin/estrogen transferred via milk to the infant is low and has no effect on the breastfed infant.

Suggested Reading:

1. Mishell DR Jr. New developments and practice guidelines: oral contraceptives and intrauterine devices. Contraception. 1998 Sep;58(3 Suppl):7S-8S. Review.
2. Vekemans M. Postpartum contraception: the lactational amenorrhea method. Eur J Contracept Reprod Health Care. 1997 Jun;2(2):105-11. Review.
3. Kubba AA. Contraception: a review. Int J Clin Pract. 1998 Mar;52(2):102-5. Review.
4. World Health Organization. Task Force on Methods for the Natural Regulation of Fertility. The WHO multinational study of breast-feeding and lactational amenorrhea. III. Pregnancy during breastfeeding. Fertil Steril 1999;72;431-440.
5. Perez A, Labbok MH, Queenan JT. Clinical study of lactational amenorrhea method for family palnning. Lancet 1992;339:968-970.
6. Dialogues In Conracception New Methods Medroxy progesterone Acetate/Estradiol Cypionate. 78; 3, 2001.
7. Valdes V, Labbak MH, Pugin E, Perez A: The efficacy of the lactational amenorrhea method (LAM) among working women. 62:5 November 2000, 217-219.
8. Kennedy KI, Labbok MH, Van Look PFA. Consensus statement on the use of breastfeeding as a family planning method. Contraception 39 (1989), pp. 55-67.
9. Nelson AL. Progestin-Only Contraceptive Methods in Breast-feeding Women. Women's Health Special Edition. Vol 1 2002 pp 25-33.
10. Guiloff E, Ibarra-Polo A, Zanartu J, et al. Effect of contraception on lactation. Am J Obstet Gynecol. 1974; 118:42-45.
11. Patel SB, Toddywalla VS, Betrabet SS, et al. At what "infant age" can levonorgestrel

contraceptives be recommended to nursing mothers? Adv Contracept. 1994; 10:249-255.

12. Virutamasen P, Leepipatpaiboon S, Kriengsinyot R, et al. Pharmacodynamic effects of depot-medroxyprogesterone acetate (DMPA) administered to lactating women on their male infants. Contraception. 1996; 54: 153-157.

13. The World Health Organization multinational study of breast-feeding and lactational amenorrhea. III. Pregnancy during breast-feeding. World Health Organization Task Forece on Methods for the Natural Regulation of Fertility. Fertil Steril 1999 Sep: 72(3): 431-40.

Cough

Principles of Therapy:

Cough is one of the most common complaints presented to physicians in the USA, accounting for 3.6% of all office visits. Cough is generally characterized by duration and etiology. The cough reflex is generally stimulated by activation of the receptors located in the tracheobronchial tree, the upper airway, and in other areas such as the sinuses, pleura, pericardium, esophagus, and other sites. The most common cause of acute cough is a viral upper respiratory infection. Occasionally, acute cough can result from inflammation and mild bronchospasm of the airways. Chronic, persistent cough should always be considered abnormal. Chronic persistent cough often occurs in smokers, asthmatics, and patients with chronic obstructive pulmonary disorder. Persistent, hacking cough can also occur following the use of drugs such as the ACE inhibitors, beta-blockers, L-dopa, environmental chemicals, or in cardiac disease. Chronic cough can occur in patients with postnatal drip, gastroesophageal reflux, asthma, and following a pulmonary infection. Treatment requires an accurate determination of etiology. Removal of offending agents such as ACE inhibitors, environmental chemicals, and allergens in the case of asthmatics, may be required in those select patients. Treatment of infectious conditions may be required in those with infected sinuses. Acute cough, particularly in cases of influenza, may require the temporary use of opioids such as codeine or dextromethorphan.

BECLOMETHASONE   AAP: Not Reviewed

> **Trade:** Vanceril, Beclovent, Beconase
> **Can/Aus/UK:** Propaderm, Vanceril, Beconase, Aldecin, Becloforte, Becotide, Beclovent
> **Specifics:** Intrapulmonary or intranasal doses are exceedingly low and penetration into milk is extremely remote. Maternal plasma levels are virtually undetectable.
> T½= 15 hours   Oral= 90%   Peak= N/A
> LRC= L2

CISAPRIDE   AAP: Compatible

> **Trade:** Propulsid
> **Can/Aus/UK:** Propulsid
> **Specifics:** Published milk levels are subclinical (6.2 μg/L).
> T½= 7-10 hours   Oral= 35-40%   Peak= 1-2 hours
> LRC= L2

CODEINE   **AAP**: Compatible

Trade: Empirin #3 # 4, Tylenol # 3 # 4
Can/Aus/UK: Paveral, Penntuss, Actacode, Codalgin, Codral, Panadeine,
Veganin, Kaodene, Teropin
Specifics: Breastmilk levels of codeine are minimal if the dose is kept less
than 60 mg.
T½= 2.9 hours   Oral= Complete   Peak= 0.5-1 hr.
LRC= L3

ESOMEPRAZOLE   **AAP**: Not Reviewed

Trade: Nexium
Can/Aus/UK: Nexium
Specifics: Esomeprazole is the L isomer of omeprazole (Prilosec). See
omeprazole below.
T½= 1 hr.   Oral= 30-40%   Peak= 0.5-3.5 hours
LRC= L3

FAMOTIDINE   **AAP**: Not Reviewed

Trade: Pepcid, Axid-Ar, Pepcid-AC
Can/Aus/UK: Pepcid, Apo-Famotidine, Novo-Famotidine, Amfamox,
Pepcidine
Specifics: Reported milk levels are very low (72 µg/L).
T½= 2.5-3.5 hours   Oral= 50%   Peak= 1-3.5 hours
LRC= L2

FLUTICASONE   **AAP**: Not Reviewed

Trade: Flonase, Flovent
Can/Aus/UK: Flovent, Flonase, Flixotide, Flixonase
Specifics: Oral and topical absorption of fluticasone is less than 2%, so it is
virtually nonabsorbed. Transfer into milk is remote. Currently available for
use in infants.
T½= 7.8 hours   Oral= <2%   Peak= 15-60 minutes
LRC= L3

NIZATIDINE   **AAP**: Not Reviewed

Trade: Axid
Can/Aus/UK: Axid, Apo-Nizatidine, Tazac
Specifics: Only minimal amounts are transferred to milk (< 0.1% of maternal
dose).
T½= 1.5 hours   Oral= 94%   Peak= 0.5-3 hours
LRC= L2

OMEPRAZOLE

AAP: Not Reviewed

Trade: Prilosec
Can/Aus/UK: Prilosec, Losec
Specifics: Omeprazole is a potent inhibitor of gastric acid secretion.   In a study of one patient receiving 20 mg omeprazole daily, the maternal serum concentration was 950 nM at 240 min. The breastmilk concentration of omeprazole began to rise minimally at 90 minutes after ingestion but peaked after 180 minutes at only 58 nM or less than 7% of the highest serum level. Omeprazole milk levels were essentially flat over 4 hours of observation. Omeprazole is extremely acid labile with a half-life of 10 minutes at pH values below 4. Virtually all omeprazole ingested via milk would probably be destroyed in the stomach of the infant prior to absorption.

T½= 1 hr.   Oral= 30-40%   Peak= 0.5-3.5 hours
LRC= L2

DEXTROMETHORPHAN

AAP: Not Reviewed

Trade: DM, Benylin, Delsym, Pertussin, Robitussin DM
Can/Aus/UK:
Specifics: Although no data is available on milk levels, its structure is similar to codeine, and it is cleared for pediatric use anyway.

T½= <4 hours   Oral= Complete   Peak= 1-2 hours
LRC= L1

Clinical Tips:

Treatment of cough depends solely on the etiology of the syndrome.   Protocols are based on the anatomy and distribution of the cough (anatomic diagnostic protocol). Acute cough of infectious etiology is generally treated with antimicrobials and antitussives such as dextromethorphan or codeine.   Of course, infections of viral etiology are only treated occasionally and with similar antitussives.   Cough of inflammatory origin such as in asthmatics is generally treated with inhaled steroids and beta-2 agonists such as albuterol.   Maternal plasma levels of these agents are generally far too low to produce clinically relevant milk levels.   Cough following postnasal drip of allergic etiology is best treated with intranasal steroids or non-sedating antihistamines.   Coughs due to gastroesophageal reflux are managed with lifestyle changes including a high protein low fat diet, not eating for 2 hours prior to lying down, elevation of the head of the bed, the use of prokinetic drugs such as cisapride or metoclopramide, or with the acid blocking drugs such as famotidine, nizatidine, or omeprazole.

Suggested Reading:

1. Lawler WR. An office approach to the diagnosis of chronic cough. Am Fam Physician. 1998 Dec;58(9):2015-22. Review.
2. Irwin RS, et al. Managing cough as a defense mechanism and as a symptom. A consensus panel report of the American College of Chest Physicians. Chest. 1998 Aug;114(2 Suppl Managing):133S-181S. Review.

Depression, Postpartum

Principles of Therapy:

Prenatal and postpartum depression generally begins 2 weeks to 6 months postpartum. Many women experience some mild letdown of mood (up to 80%) following delivery refered to as post-partum "blues". This is frequently experienced days 3-6 after delivery and is generally transient requiring supportive therapy. In some (10-15%) the symptoms are much more severe and persistent and may warrant therapy. Symptoms include: hypomania, obsessive thoughts about harming the infant, sleep deprivation, volatility of behavior, weight loss, suicide ideation, and others. Predisposing factors for post-partum depression include a prior history of depressive illness and adolescence (30% risk of depression) whereas the patient who has previously experienced post-partum depression has a recurrence risk as high as 70%. Bipolar disorders are distinguished by both manic and depressive symptoms. Mania is characterized by elation with hyperactivity, flight of ideas, over enthusiasm, easy distractibility, and insomnia. With virtually all of the following medications, onset is rather slow, up to 3-4 weeks. The SSRI family appear to work somewhat faster than the tricyclic family, but this varies.

AMITRIPTYLINE   **AAP**: May be of concern

Trade: Elavil, Endep
Can/Aus/UK: Apo-Amitriptyline, Elavil, Novo-Tryptin, Amitrol, Endep, Mutabon D, Tryptanol, Domical, Lentizol
Specifics: Levels in breastmilk are reported to be quite small. Numerous studies indicate minimal effects on nursing infant.
T½= 31-46 hours   Oral= Complete   Peak= 2-4 hours
LRC= L2

AMOXAPINE   **AAP**: May be of concern

Trade: Asendin
Can/Aus/UK:
Specifics: Following a dose of 250 mg/day, milk levels of amoxapine were less than 20µg/L and 113µg/L of the active metabolite. Milk levels of active metabolite varied from 113 to 168µg/L in two other milk samples. Milk levels are generally less than 20% of the maternal plasma level.
T½= 8 hours(parent)   Oral= 18-54%   Peak= 2 hours
LRC= L2

BUPROPION   **AAP**: Not Reviewed

Trade: Wellbutrin, Zyban
Can/Aus/UK:
Specifics: While this drug has a high milk/plasma ratio, it is not detectable in the infants plasma. Hence the absolute dose via milk is very low. May lower seizure threshold so do not use in patients or breastfeeding mothers whose infants suffer from seizure disorders.
T½= 8-24 hours   Oral= N/A   Peak= 2 hours
LRC= L3

CLOMIPRAMINE   **AAP**: Compatible

Trade: Anafranil
Can/Aus/UK: Anafranil, Apo-Clomipramine, Placil
Specifics: May be especially useful for panic disorders, or obsessive-compulsive disorder.
T½= 19-37 hours   Oral= Complete   Peak= N/A
LRC= L2

DESIPRAMINE   **AAP**: May be of concern

Trade: Pertofrane, Norpramin
Can/Aus/UK: Norpramin, Pertofrane,Novo-Desipramine, Pertofran
Specifics: In one case report, a mother taking 200 mg of desipramine at bedtime had milk/plasma ratios of 0.4 to 0.9 with milk levels ranging between 17-35 µg/L.
T½= 7-60 hours   Oral= 90%   Peak= 4-6 hours
LRC= L2

DOTHIEPIN   **AAP**: May be of concern

Trade: Prothiaden
Can/Aus/UK:
Specifics: Dothiepin appears in breastmilk in a concentration of 11 µg/L following a dose of 75 mg/day, while the maternal plasma level was 33µg/L. If the infant ingests 150 mL/kg/day of milk, the total daily dose of dothiepin ingested by the infant in this case would be approximately 1.65 µg/kg/day, approximately 1/650th of the adult dose.
T½= 14.4-23.9 hours   Oral= 30%   Peak= 3 hours
LRC= L2

FLUOXETINE   AAP: May be of concern

Trade: Prozac
Can/Aus/UK: Prozac, Apo-Fluoxetine, Novo-Fluoxetine, Lovan, Zactin
Specifics: Fluoxetine, and its metabolite norfluoxetine, have very long half-lives. Several reports indicate high plasma levels in some infants. Symptoms reported include colic, insomnia, tremors, crying, and one case of coma. Use during pregnancy, followed by use during lactation may be inadvisable. Use cautiously in mothers with premature or newborns infants. Its use in older infants (> 4 months) is probably less risky.
T½= 2-3 days(fluoxetine)   Oral= 100%   Peak= 1.5 - 12 hours
LRC= L2 in older infants
           L3 if used in neonatal peiod

CITALOPRAM   AAP: Not Reviewed

Trade: Celexa
Can/Aus/UK:
Specifics: The newest SSRI, citalopram,   enters milk in low levels. Estimated daily intake for an infant would be approximately 4.3-14.6 µg/kg/day. This would be less than 5.9% of the weight-adjusted maternal dose. No untoward effects were reported in breastfed infants.
T½= 36 hours   Oral= 80%   Peak= 2-4 hours
LRC= L3

FLUVOXAMINE   AAP: Not Reviewed

Trade: Luvox
Can/Aus/UK: Luvox, Apo-Fluvoxamine, Alti-Fluvoxamine, Luvox, Faverin, Floxyfral, Myroxim
Specifics: In a case report of one 23 year old mother and following a dose of 100 mg twice daily for 2 weeks, the maternal plasma level of fluvoxamine base was 0.31 mg/Liter and the milk concentration was 0.09 mg/Liter. The authors reported a theoretical dose to infant of 0.0104 mg/kg/day of fluvoxamine, which is only 0.5% of the maternal dose.
T½= 15.6 hours   Oral= 53%   Peak= 3-8 hours
LRC= L2

IMIPRAMINE   AAP: May be of concern

Trade: Tofranil, Janimine
Can/Aus/UK: Apo-Imipramine, Impril, Novo-Pramine, Melipramine, Tofranil
Specifics: Dose via milk is low and is estimated to be from 20-200 µg per day. No untoward effects noted in breastfed infants.

T½= 8-16 hours   Oral= 90%   Peak= 1-2 hours
LRC= L2

NORTRIPTYLINE   AAP: Not Reviewed

Trade: Aventyl, Pamelor
Can/Aus/UK: Aventyl, Norventyl, Apo-Nortriptyline, Allegron
Specifics: Milk levels of nortriptyline are low to undetectable. No untoward effects have been reported in several studies.

T½= 16-90 hours   Oral= 51%   Peak= 7-8.5 hours
LRC= L2

PAROXETINE   AAP: Not Reviewed

Trade: Paxil
Can/Aus/UK: Paxil, Aropax 20, Seroxat
Specifics: In a recent study of 16 mothers by Stowe,   paroxetine levels in milk were low and varied   according to maternal dose.   Milk/plasma ratios varied from 0.056 to 1.3.   Milk levels ranged from approximately 17 µg/L, 45 µg/L, 70 µg/L,   92 µg/L and 101 µg/L in mothers receiving a dose of 10, 20, 30, 40, and   50 mg/day respectively.   Levels of paroxetine were below the limit of detection (< 2 ng/mL) in all 16 infants.   Numerous other studies generally conclude that paroxetine can be considered relatively safe for breastfeeding infants as the absolute dose transferred is quite low.   Plasma levels in the infant were generally undetectable.   Recent data suggests that a neonatal withdrawal syndrome may occur in newborns exposed in utero to paroxetine.

T½= 21 hours   Oral= Complete   Peak= 5-8 hours
LRC= L2

SERTRALINE   AAP: Not Reviewed

Trade: Zoloft
Can/Aus/UK: Zoloft, Lustral
Specifics: At this time, more than 60 breastfeeding infants have been studied following maternal use of sertraline. Thus far, no untoward effects have been reported, and in almost all cases, no medication was detectable in the plasma compartment of the infant.

T½= 26-65 hours   Oral= Complete   Peak= 7-8 hours
LRC= L2

TRAZODONE   **AAP**: May be of concern

Trade: Desyrel
Can/Aus/UK:
Specifics: In six mothers who received a single 50 mg dose, the milk/plasma ratio averaged 0.14.   Peak milk concentrations occurred at 2 hours   On a weight basis, an adult would receive 0.77 mg/kg whereas a breastfeeding infant, using this data, would consume only 0.005 mg/kg. About 0.6 % of the maternal dose was ingested by the infant.
T½= 4-9 hours   Oral= 65%   Peak= 1-2 hours
LRC= L2

VENLAFAXINE   **AAP**: Not Reviewed

Trade: Effexor
Can/Aus/UK: Effexor
Specifics: The mean total infant dose was 7.6% of the maternal weight-adjusted dose. The metabolite of venlafaxine (but not venlafaxine) was detected in all three infants at low levels. The infants were healthy and showed no acute adverse effects.
T½= 5 hours(venlafaxine)   Oral= 92%   Peak= N/A
LRC= L3

Clinical Tips:

Current studies now suggest that infants of depressed mothers may not have normal neurobehavioral development at one year.   Treatment largely depends on severity and a risk vs. benefit assessment.   Many studies show minimal to no effect of the tricyclics on infants or their neurobehavioral development.   Of the newer SSRIs, sertraline(Zoloft) appears safest, with more than 60 mother-infants pairs studied to date and no untoward effects noted in these studies.   Other SSRIs such as paroxetine and venlafaxine have been studied and found without untoward effects on the infant. Although somewhat controversial, fluoxetine should be used with some caution particularly in the newborn period.   While many mothers have breastfed while using fluoxetine, numerous reports both published and via personal communication suggest that this product can produce symptoms including colic, sedation, insomnia, hyperthermia, and even coma.   Using fluoxetine early postpartum in mothers of premature or newborn infants may be risky, particularly if the mother has received fluoxetine during pregnancy.   In these cases conversion to another SSRI is suggested.   Treatment of mothers 3 or more months postpartum with fluoxetine may be less problematic as the infant is more able to eliminate this product effectively.

Recently several cases of neonatal withdrawal syndrome (early postpartum) have been reported in infants of mothers who ingested the shorter half-life SSRIs such as paroxetine, sertraline (while pregnant) and even one case of fluoxetine. These symptoms generally arise early postpartum, such as 24-72 hours. Neonatal withdrawal symptoms include irritability, constant crying, shivering, increased tonus, eating and sleeping difficulties, and convulsions. These early symptoms of withdrawal should not be confused with similar symptoms seen in reported cases of fluoxetine toxicity, which generally included hyperthermia. The SSRI withdrawal symptoms seen early postpartum generally resolve without treatment within a few days. Breastfeeding should continue in these cases.

Suggested Reading:

1.   Cooper PJ, et al. Postnatal depression. Cooper PJ, et al. BMJ. 1998 Jun 20;316(7148):1884-6. Review.
2.   Nonacs R, et al. Postpartum mood disorders: diagnosis and treatment guidelines. J Clin Psychiatry. 1998;59 Suppl 2:34-40. Review.
3.   Pariser SF, et al. Postpartum mood disorders: clinical perspectives. J Womens Health. 1997 Aug;6(4):421-34. Review.
4.   Susman JL. Postpartum depressive disorders. J Fam Pract. 1996 Dec;
5.   Nordeng H, et.al. Neonatal withdrawal syndrome after in utero exposure to selective serotonin reuptake inhibitors. Acta Paediatr 2001; 90(3):288-91.

Diabetes Mellitus

Principles of Therapy:

Diabetes mellitus is a heterogenous group of disorders characterized by abnormal insulin secretion, lipid and carbohydrate metabolism. It is also the most common endocrine disorder affecting women in pregnancy. Over 90% of diabetics have non-insulin dependent diabetes (NIDDM), while 5-10% have insulin-dependent diabetes (IDDM). The hallmark of IDDM is the loss of the pancreatic beta cells and their source of insulin. Exogenous insulin repletion is the only source of treatment. In IDDM mothers, exogenous insulin does not transfer into human milk; its molecular weight is simply too large to permit entry into the milk compartment. Hence, insulin treatment in IDDM patients is not a contraindication to breastfeeding. But the vast majority of patients are NIDDM who may require oral antidiabetic agents. Unfortunately, this area of breastfeeding pharmacology is poorly studied and the number of medications that have been studied in breastfeeding mothers is limited. Gestational diabetes requiring medication is usually treated with insulin and will not require extended therapy beyond pregnancy unless the underlying problem was truly undiagnosed pre-existing diabetes. However, approximately 50% of women with gestational diabetes will go on to develop overt diabetes within 20 years. All infants of diabetic mothers, regardless of type, are at increased risk of hypoglycemia at birth and glucose testing of the infant within 30 minutes of birth is recommended

CHLORPROPAMIDE   AAP: Not Reviewed

Trade: Diabenese
Can/Aus/UK: Apo-Chlorpropamide, Diabinese, Novopropamide, Melitase
Specifics: Levels in milk are approximately 5 mg/liter of milk. These are probably too low to produce hypoglycemia in infants.
T½= 33 hours   Oral= Complete   Peak= 3-6 hours
LRC= L3

INSULIN   AAP: Not Reviewed

Trade: Humulin
Can/Aus/UK: Novolin, Humulin, Humalog, Iletin, Mixtard, Protaphane, Monotard
Specifics: Insulin is too large in molecular weight to enter milk. Levels are nil.
T½= N/A   Oral= 0%   Peak= N/A
LRC= L1

METFORMIN
AAP: Not Reviewed

Trade: Glucophage
Can/Aus/UK: Glucophage, Gen-Metformin, Glycon, Diabex, Diaformin, Diguanil
Specifics: In a preliminary study of 5 women who received 500 mg three times daily, milk levels were extremely low. While the average milk/plasma ratio was 0.34, the average dose to the infant was 0.0405 mg/kg/d or 0.26% of the weight-adjusted maternal dose. In this study, no adverse effects were noted in any infant.
T½= 6.2 hours(plasma)   Oral= 50%   Peak= 2.75 hours
LRC= L3

TOLBUTAMIDE
AAP: Compatible

Trade: Oramide, Orinase
Can/Aus/UK: Apo-Tolbutamide, Mobenol, Novo-Butamide, Orinase, Rastinon, Glyconon
Specifics: Milk levels are very low, only 3 to 18 µg/liter of milk.
T½= 4.5-6.5 hours   Oral= Complete   Peak= 3.5 hours
LRC= L3

ACARBOSE
AAP: Not Reviewed

Trade: Precose
Can/Aus/UK:
Specifics: Acarbose is not bioavailable but is metabolized in the GI tract to a number of inactive metabolites, some of which are absorbed systemically. The metabolites would not likely enter milk to any degree.
T½= < 2 hours   Oral= 0.7- 2%   Peak= N/A
LRC= L3

Clinical Tips:
Insulin, due to its large molecular weight (>6000), does not enter milk in clinically relevant amounts, so it can be readily used in breastfeeding mothers with IDDM. Of the sulfonylureas, only tolbutamide and chlorpropamide have been measured in human milk. The levels of these two sulfonylureas were quite small and are probably subclinical. Unfortunately, the newer second generation sulfonylureas (e.g. glipizide, glimepiride, glyburide) have not been studied. While one cannot say for sure that they are safe, no reports of hypoglycemic infants have been found. Metformin transfer into human milk is poor. In a study of 7 women receiving 1500 mg daily, the average milk concentration was only 0.27 mg/L. The absolute infant dose from breastmilk averaged 0.04 mg/kg/day and the mean relative infant dose was only 0.28% of the maternal dose.

Metformin levels in the plasma of the studied infants were very low or undetectable.

It is unlikely the amount transferred to an infant would be clinically relevant. Of these hypoglycemic agents, metformin has a number of benefits and is often a first choice drug in women with polycystic ovary disease and now NIDDM. Its use in women with polycystic ovary syndrome is common and growing, and this has increased it use in pregnant and postpartum breastfeeding women. The fact that it is weight-negative, thus inducing weight loss in many patients is advantageous. The newer thiazolidinediones such as rosiglitazone(Avandia) and pioglitazone(Actos) have yet to be studied in breastfeeding mothers but maternal plasma levels are quite low, and their protein binding is very high(> 99%) thus milk levels would probably be quite low although this is only theoretical. The alpha-glucosidate inhibitors such as acarbose (Precose) and miglitol (Glyset) act by slowing the absorption of carbohydrates in the intestine. Interestingly, they are poorly bioavailable and stay in the gut. It is not at all likely they would ever transfer into milk and affect an infant. But this has yet to be studied in breastfeeding mothers.

A risk-vs-benefit assessment may assist the clinician prior to its use in breastfeeding mothers. It is important to remember that gestational diabetics often revert to normal soon after delivery, suggesting that a few months of insulin therapy or metformin if it works would be ideal for continuing breastfeeding.

Suggested Reading:

1. Standl E. Overview of the management of type 2 diabetes. Diabetes Metab Rev. 1998 Sep;14 Suppl 1:S13-7. Review.
2. Mayfield J. Diagnosis and classification of diabetes mellitus: new criteria. Am Fam Physician. 1998 Oct 15;58(6):1355-62, 1369-70. Review.
3. Hague WM. Drugs in pregnancy. Endocrine disease (including diabetes). Best Pract Res Clin Obstet Gynaecol. 2001 Dec;15(6):877-89. Review.
4. Hale, TW, Kristensen JH, Hackett LP, Kohan R. and Ilett KF. Transfer of metformin into human milk. In Publication, 2002.
5. Drexler AJ, Robertson C. Type 2 diabetes. How new insights, new drugs are changing clinical practice. Geriatrics. 2001 Jun;56(6):20-4, 32-3. Review.

Fever

Principles of Therapy:

Fever is a common manifestation of numerous medical conditions, both serious and minor. Fever is generally protective, and only in rare conditions, is treatment actually required. There are multiple causes of hyperthermia which include: infectious disease, chemicals such as salicylates, anticholinergics, stimulants, anesthetics, dehydration, elevated environmental temperatures, excessive body wrapping, excessive exercise, head trauma, malignancies, hyperthyroidism, etc. Fever is in many instances beneficial, including stimulation of the immune system, accelerated destruction of viruses, bacteria, and some malignancies. The relationship between excessive fever and brain damage is weak, and most data suggests otherwise. Treatment of fever solely depends on determining the etiology of the syndrome, whether infectious, chemical, or environmental. Appropriate treatment of fever in a breastfeeding woman will depend on treatment of the specific underlying instigating cause.

ACETAMINOPHEN
AAP: Compatible

Trade: Tempra, Tylenol, Paracetamol
Can/Aus/UK: Apo-Acetaminophen, Tempra, Tylenol, Paracetamol, Panadol, Dymadon, Calpol
Specifics: Only minimal amounts are secreted in milk.
T1/2= 2 hours   Oral= >85%   Peak= 0.5-2 hours
LRC= L1

ASPIRIN
AAP: May be of concern

Trade: Aspirin, Ecotrin, Excedrin
Can/Aus/UK: Ecotrin
Specifics: Aspirin levels in human milk are exceedingly low. Occasional use in breastfeeding mothers is not absolutely contraindicated. It should never be used when the infant is sick or febrile, due to its relationship with Reye's syndrome.
T½= 2.5-7 hours   Oral= 80-100%   Peak= 1-2 hours
LRC= L3

IBUPROFEN
AAP: Compatible

Trade: Advil, Nuprin, Motrin, Pediaprofen
Can/Aus/UK: Actiprofen, Advil, Amersol, Motrin, ACT-3, Brufen, Nurofen, Rafen
Specifics: Ibuprofen is an ideal NSAID for breastfeeding mother due to

short half-life and minimal breastmilk levels.

T1/2= 1.8-2.5 hours   Oral= 80%   Peak= 1-2 hours

LRC= L1

Clinical Tips:

Non-drug therapies of fever include: hydration, removing of excess clothing, avoidance of exercise, removal from excessive environmental temperatures, and bathing in lukewarm water (not ice water or alcohol). Cooling blankets may be used in an inpatient setting. Topical alcohol is absorbed through the skin, and can induce a chemical pneumonitis or ketosis. Alcohol should be avoided. Acetaminophen is an ideal antipyretic when administered in proper doses. Except in rare circumstances with severe hepatotoxicity, normal therapeutic doses appear to be very safe. Doses in adults are 325 – 650 mg every 3-4 hours. Ibuprofen has recently become very popular as an antipyretic. Therapeutic doses of ibuprofen produce a more rapid fall in temperature, and a longer duration (5-8 hours) than with acetaminophen. This effect is more evident upon initial use, and may not sustain itself after repeated use. Ibuprofen is the safest NSAID for use in breastfeeding mothers, as milk levels are very small. Ibuprofen should not be used in patients with gastric ulcers, nor in a mother in her third trimester (closure of ductus arteriosus), and only cautiously in asthmatic patients. Although aspirin levels in milk are low, the fear of Reye's syndrome has stopped their use in pediatrics, and is of theoretical concern in breastfeeding mothers.

Suggested Reading:

1. Kluger MJ, et al. Role of fever in disease. Ann N Y Acad Sci. 1998 Sep 29;856:224-33. Review.
2. Mackowiak PA, et al. Benefits and risks of antipyretic therapy. Ann N Y Acad Sci. 1998 Sep 29;856:214-23. Review.
3. Mackowiak PA. Concepts of fever. Arch Intern Med. 1998 Sep 28;158(17):1870-81. Review.

Gastroesophageal Reflux

Principles of Therapy:

Gastroesophageal reflux disease (GERD) is the most common disorder of the esophagus. GERD arises following recurrent regurgitation of gastric acids past the lower esophageal sphincter and into the lower esophagus. The major determinant of esophageal symptoms and damage is prolonged contact of refluxed gastric acid with the esophageal epithelium. Symptoms occur most often at night, when the patient is recumbent. Gastric acids can easily pass the lower esophageal sphincter, and enter the esophagus while the patient is horizontal. Medical therapy alleviates many of the symptoms, but GERD should be considered a chronic condition, especially in patients with inflammatory esophagitis. Treatment consists of the use of antacids, acid blocking agents, and occasionally the prokinetic drugs (cisapride, metoclopramide).

CISAPRIDE
AAP: Compatible

Trade: Propulsid
Can/Aus/UK: Propulsid, Prepulsid
Specifics: While not available in the US, it is still used in other regions. Published milk levels are subclinical (6.2 µg/L).
T½= 7-10 hours   Oral= 35-40%   Peak= 1-2 hours
LRC= L2

ESOMEPRAZOLE
AAP: Not Reviewed

Trade: Nexium
Can/Aus/UK: Nexium
Specifics: Esomeprazole is the L isomer of omeprazole (Prilosec). See omeprazole below.
T½= 1 hr.   Oral= 30-40%   Peak= 0.5-3.5 hours
LRC= L3

FAMOTIDINE
AAP: Not Reviewed

Trade: Pepcid, Axid-AR, Pepcid-AC
Can/Aus/UK: Pepcid, Apo-Famotidine, Novo-Famotidine, Amfamox, Pepcidine
Specifics: Reported milk levels are very low (72µg/L).
T½= 2.5-3.5 hours   Oral= 50%   Peak= 1-3.5 hours
LRC= L2

NIZATIDINE
AAP: Not Reviewed

Trade: Axid
Can/Aus/UK: Axid, Apo-Nizatidine, Tazac
Specifics: Only minimal amounts are transferred to milk (< 0.1% of maternal dose).
T½= 1.5 hours   Oral= 94%   Peak= 0.5-3 hours
LRC= L2

OMEPRAZOLE
AAP: Not Reviewed

Trade: Prilosec
Can/Aus/UK: Prilosec, Losec
Specifics: Omeprazole is a potent inhibitor of gastric acid secretion. In a study of one patient receiving 20 mg omeprazole daily, the maternal serum concentration was 950 nM at 240 min. The breastmilk concentration of omeprazole began to rise minimally at 90 minutes after ingestion, but peaked after 180 minutes at only 58 nM, or less than 7% of the highest serum level. Omeprazole milk levels were essentially flat over 4 hours of observation. Omeprazole is extremely acid labile with a half-life of 10 minutes at pH values below 4. Virtually all omeprazole ingested via milk would be destroyed in the stomach of the infant prior to absorption.
T½= 1 hour   Oral= 30-40%   Peak= 0.5-3.5 hours
LRC= L2

RANITIDINE
AAP: Not Reviewed

Trade: Zantac
Can/Aus/UK: Apo-Ranitidine, Novo-Ranidine, Zantac, Nu-Ranit
Specifics: While the milk/plasma ratio is quite high, the absolute dose to the infant is quite low. Following a dose of 150 mg for four doses, the concentrations in breastmilk were 0.72, 2.6, and 1.5 mg/L at 1.5, 5.5 and 12 hours respectively. Using this data, an infant consuming 1 L of milk daily would ingest less than 2.6 mg/24 hours. This amount is quite small considering the pediatric dose currently recommended is 2-4 mg/kg/24 hours.
T½= 2-3 hours   Oral= 50%   Peak= 1-3 hours
LRC= L2

SUCRALFATE
AAP: Not Reviewed

Trade: Carafate
Can/Aus/UK: Sulcrate, Novo-Sucralate, Nu-Sucralfate, Carafate, SCF, Ulcyte, Antepsin
Specifics: Sucralfate acts topically to cover the mucosal lining of the esophagus, stomach, and duodenum. Less than 5% is absorbed and it is

unlikely to penetrate milk.

T½= N/A   Oral= < 5%   Peak= N/A

LRC= L2

Clinical Tips:

Initial therapy of GERD is comprised of antacids or the H2 receptor blockers (e.g. famotidine, ranitidine). Of the antacids, Gaviscon (alginic acids and antacids) is quite popular as it floats on the stomach contents, thus covering the lower esophageal sphincter. However, in more difficult cases the H2 blockers are quite effective. Famotidine and nizatidine produce only minimal levels in breastmilk and are probably preferred over ranitidine. However, ranitidine levels in breastmilk are probably too low to produce a clinical effect. In more severe cases of GERD, omeprazole is preferred, as it produces almost complete blockage of acid secretion for long periods (24 hours). A recent study suggests milk levels are flat during the day and also minimal. Any omeprazole present in milk would be instantly destroyed in the infant's stomach prior to absorption. Esomeprazole (Nexium) is the active ingredient of omeprazole(Prilosec) and should be safe for use in breastfeeding mothers. Sucralfate is the aluminum salt of sucrose octasulfate. It acts topically, binding to acid, pepsin, and bile on the stomach or esophageal lining. None would be expected to enter milk. Of the prokinetic agents, cisapride is an obvious first choice in GERD patients when needed. The amount of cisapride in milk is only 6.2 µg/Liter. When compared to the clinical dose used in infants (0.3 mg/Kg) the amount in milk is minimal.

Suggested Reading:

1.   Navaratnam RM, et al.Gastro-oesophageal reflux: the disease of the millennium. Hosp Med. 1998 Aug;59(8):646-9. Review.
2.   Mujica VR, et al. Recognizing atypical manifestations of GERD. Asthma, chest pain, and otolaryngologic disorders may be due to reflux. Postgrad Med. 1999 Jan;105(1):53-5, 60, 63-6. Review.
3.   Dent J. Gastro-oesophageal reflux disease. Digestion. 1998 Aug;59(5):433-45. Review.
4.   Lee JM, et al. Trends in the management of gastro-oesophageal reflux disease. Postgrad Med J. 1998 Mar;74(869):145-50. Review.

Glaucoma

Principles of Therapy:

Glaucoma is a group of ocular diseases that have in common an optic neuropathy that causes visual loss. Elevated intraocular pressure is the most important, and only modifiable risk factor for glaucoma. Treatment for the various types of glaucoma are specific and the essential diagnosis of the mechanism of glaucoma is required. Acute (Angle-closure) glaucoma occurs most commonly in older patients with acute onset pain, profound visual loss, red eye, steamy cornea, and dilated pupil. Primary acute angle-closure glaucoma is almost always associated with pupillary dilation from setting in a darkened environment, at times of stress, from pharmacologic mydriasis during eye examinations, or from systemic anticholinergic medications(atropine-like). Open-angle glaucoma on the other hand has an insidious onset, generally in older age groups. Symptoms are minimal if present at all, with gradual loss of peripheral vision of a period of years. In open-angle glaucoma the intraocular pressure is consistently elevated. Over months and years, this ultimately results in optic atrophy with loss of vision. In the USA, it is estimated that 1-2% of people over 40 have glaucoma. About 90% are open-angle glaucoma. Unfortunately, breastfeeding studies of the agents used to treat glaucoma are poor and few. The medications below are primarily used to reduce intraocular pressures by one of several mechanisms.

ACETAZOLAMIDE   AAP: Compatible

Trade: Dazamide, Diamox
Can/Aus/UK: Acetazolam, Apo-Acetazolamide, Diamox
Specifics: Levels in milk are minimal although maternal side effect profile is significant including blood dyscrasia.
T½= 2.4-5.8 hours   Oral= Complete   Peak= 1-3 hours
LRC= L2

TIMOLOL   AAP: Compatible

Trade: Blocadren
Can/Aus/UK: Apo-Timol, Timoptic, Novo-Timol, Tenopt, Timpilo, Betim, Blocadren, Timoptol
Specifics: Two studies show levels in milk are low and subclinical.
T½= 4 hours   Oral= 50%   Peak= 1-2 hours
LRC= L2

LATANOPROST   AAP: Not Reviewed

Trade: Xalatan
Can/Aus/UK: Xalatan
Specifics: No data is available, but systemic absorption and half-life (17 minutes) is minimal. First pass liver uptake is high. Unlikely to enter milk.
T½= < 30 minutes   Oral= Nil   Peak= < 1 hour
LRC= L3

PILOCARPINE   AAP: Not Reviewed

Trade: Isopto Carpine, Pilocar, Akarpine
Can/Aus/UK:
Specifics: No studies are available, but the half-life is brief and the systemic effects following ophthalmic use are minimal.
T½= 0.76-1.55 hours   Oral= N/A   Peak= 1.25 hours
LRC= L3

Clinical Tips:

The topical beta-blockers, timolol, levobunolol, and betaxolol are effective ocular hypotensives and work by decreasing the production of aqueous humor. Systemic absorption via absorption by the nasal mucosa is known and can be reduced by digital occlusion of the nasolacrimal drainage system for several minutes following installation of the drops. Reported side effects associated with topical beta-blockers include bronchospasm and shortness of breath, depression and fatigue, confusion; impotence; hair loss, heart failure; and bradycardia. Several studies of timolol show no effect on nursing infants. Betaxolol may be a second choice following one report of side effects in a nursing infant.

Oral carbonic anhydrase inhibitors (eg, acetazolamide, methazolamide) are effective in lowering intraocular pressure IOP. However, their side effect include anorexia, depression, kidney stones, fatigue, abnormalities in serum electrolytes, and blood dyscrasias which often limit their usefulness. They are probably not suitable for long-term use in breastfeeding mothers.

Although no data are available, latanoprost(Xalatan) could probably be useful in breastfeeding mothers as its plasma half-life (17 minutes) is extremely brief and its poor systemic bioavailability is unlikely to produce clinically relevant levels in milk. A topical prostaglandin, latanoprost in a single daily application, effectively lowers intraocular pressure for 24 hours. It is generally well tolerated with few systemic side effects. The major ocular side effects are increased pigmentation of the iris, particularly in hazel-colored irises, and possible worsening of uveitis. A new prostaglandin F2-alpha analogue, travoprost (Travatan) with ocular hypotensive activity also produces minimal plasma levels and has a brief half-life of less than 30 minutes. While the manufacturer suggests it is present in rodent milk, no human data are available. It is not likely to be orally bioavailable in an infant.

Other agents such as the organophosphates which include echothiophate, have not been studied in breastfeeding women but should be used with caution as they irreversibly inhibit acetylcholine esterase and can produce systemic effects.

Suggested Reading:

1. Dreyer EB, et al. New perspectives on glaucoma. JAMA. 1999 Jan 27;281(4):306-8. Review.
2. Alward WL. Medical management of glaucoma. N Engl J Med. 1998 Oct 29;339(18):1298-307. Review.
3. Podolsky MM. Exposing glaucoma. Primary care physicians are instrumental in early detection. Postgrad Med. 1998 May;103(5):131-6, 142-3, 147-8. Review.
4. Frishman WH, Kowalski M, Nagnur S, Warshafsky S, Sica D. Cardiovascular considerations in using topical, oral, and intravenous drugs for the treatment of glaucoma and ocular hypertension: focus on beta-adrenergic blockade. Heart Dis. 2001 Nov-Dec;3(6):386-97. Review.

Headache

Principles of Therapy:

Headache is such a common term, and can occur for so many reasons that it is difficult to properly evaluate. Although underlying pathology such as brain tumor is very uncommon, it is important to remember that over 33% of brain tumor patients present with headache. The choice of therapy largely depends on frequency, intensity, site, and preexisting conditions (pregnancy, breastfeeding, etc) in the patient. For the purpose of this category, migraine and cluster headaches are presented under their own sections later.

ACETAMINOPHEN   AAP: Compatible

Trade: Tempra, Tylenol, Paracetamol
Can/Aus/UK: Apo-Acetaminophen, Tempra, Tylenol, Paracetamol, Panadol, Dymadon, Calpol
Specifics: Only minimal amounts are secreted in milk.
T½= 2 hours   Oral= >85%   Peak= 0.5-2 hours
LRC= L1

ASPIRIN   AAP: May be of concern

Trade: Aspirin, Ecotrin, Excedrin
Can/Aus/UK: Aspirin, Ecotrin
Specifics: Aspirin levels in human milk are exceedingly low. Occasional use in breastfeeding mothers is not absolutely contraindicated. It should never be used when the infant is sick or febrile, due to its relationship with Reye's syndrome.
T½= 2.5-7 hours   Oral= 80-100%   Peak= 1-2 hours
LRC= L3

CODEINE   AAP: Compatible

Trade: Empirin #3 # 4, Tylenol # 3 # 4
Can/Aus/UK: Paveral, Penntuss, Actacode, Codalgin, Codral, Panadeine, Veganin, Kaodene, Teropin
Specifics: Breastmilk levels of codeine are minimal, if the dose is kept less than 60 mg.
T½= 2.9 hours   Oral= Complete   Peak= 0.5-1 hr.
LRC= L3

IBUPROFEN   AAP: Compatible

Trade: Advil, Nuprin, Motrin, Pediaprofen
Can/Aus/UK: Actiprofen, Advil, Amersol, Motrin, ACT-3, Brufen, Nurofen, Rafen
Specifics: Ibuprofen is an ideal NSAID for breastfeeding mother due to short half-life and minimal breastmilk levels.
T½= 1.8-2.5 hours   Oral= 80%   Peak= 1-2 hour
LRC= L1

NAPROXEN   AAP: Compatible

Trade: Anaprox, Naprosyn, Naproxen, Aleve
Can/Aus/UK: Anaprox, Apo-Naproxen, Naprosyn, Naxen, Inza, Naprosyn, Proxen SR, Synflex
Specifics: Naproxen is a longer half-life NSAID and as such is should not be used for long periods in order to prevent buildup in the infant. Infrequent use is not contraindicated, particularly with older infants.
T½= 12-15 hours   Oral= 74-99%   Peak= 2-4 hours
LRC= L3
        L4 for chronic use

Clinical Tips:
Acetaminophen, particularly early postpartum, is the ideal choice for analgesia. It does not affect clotting, nor does it transfer to the infant in clinically relevant doses. Ibuprofen is an ideal analgesic as well for breastfeeding mothers because the milk levels are so low, its half-life is short, and it is cleared for use in pediatric patients. It has been commonly used in postpartum women with minimal side effects for quite some time. While using opiates for headaches is not always advisable, codeine is not contraindicated in breastfeeding women. It is the most common analgesic used for postpartum pain management. While naproxen is not definitely contraindicated, its use should be limited to infrequent and brief periods.

Suggested Reading:
1.   Jackson CM. Effective headache management. Strategies to help patients gain control over pain. Postgrad Med. 1998 Nov;104(5):133-6, 139-40, 143-7. Review.
2.   Horne M. Treating headaches. A conceptual framework. Aust Fam Physician. 1998 Jul;27(7):579-86. Review.
3.   Sharfman M. Update on headache. Compr Ther. 1998 Apr;24(4):194-7. Review.

Hypertension

Principles of Therapy:

Non-Puerperal Hypertension:

Primary or essential hypertension is of unknown etiology. Generally, increased total peripheral resistance (TPR), or increased cardiac output lead to elevated blood pressure. The choice of antihypertensive largely rests on the primary source of the syndrome which could include elevated sympathetic output, elevated plasma volume, elevated renin secretions by the kidney, or other etiologies. Therapy is largely guided by the source of pathology, age and clinical condition of patient. Initial therapy for non-puerperal hypertension should include dietary changes and modification of life style such as weight loss for obese patients, smoking cessation, restriction of alcohol and sodium intake and exercise. If these methods are unsuccessful after 3 months or the clinical situation otherwise warrants medication then pharmacologic agents are begun. Beta-blockers are indicated for younger patients, patients with arrhythmias, angina pectoris, early onset hypertension, and post-MI patients. Diuretics (thiazides) are primarily indicated for black patients, older, obese, edematous patients and individuals subject to congestive heart failure. Calcium channel blockers (CCB) are quite controversial. They were previously indicated primarily for older patients, and those with angina, arrhythmias, congestive heart failure, and SVT. However, some current studies show increased morbidity with the CCB agents.

Gestational Hypertension:

Hypertension during pregnancy may be either chronic hypertension which either continues or is diagnosed during pregnancy or hypertension specifically related to pregnancy such as pre-eclampsia. First line management of chronic hypertension during pregnancy will often employ methyldopa or labetalol. If effective these may be continued during the lactational period. Hydralazine has a long history of safety and efficacy in pre-eclampsia and postpartum hypertension. Although the ACE inhibitors are quite safe for adult patients, their use during pregnancy and the post-partum period is hazardous. Infants are ultra sensitive to the ACE family and caution is urged. Older infants (> 1 month) can probably handle the small amounts present in milk. ACE inhibitors are contraindicated during the second and third trimester of pregnancy due to an association with adverse fetal/neonatal outcomes including under-developed calvarium, renal failure, oligohydramnios, fetal growth restriction, renal dysgenesis, pulmonary hypoplasia and fetal and neonatal death. Atenolol is also discouraged for use during pregnancy due to potential concern for fetal growth restriction though this information is less conclusive. Women with pre-ecclampsia will require the use of magnesium sulfate for seizure prophylaxis during the peri-partum period.(See seizure disorders). In this setting, treatement of hypertension depends on severity but frequently will be accomplished by hydralazine or labetalol. Diuretics are rarely useful in the management of pre-ecclampsia.

METHYLDOPA   **AAP**: Compatible
> **Trade:**   Aldomet
> **Can/Aus/UK:** Aldomet, Apo-Methlydopa, Dopamet, Novo-Medopa, Aldopren, Hydopa, Nudopa
> ***Specifics:***   Reported milk levels are quite low in over 9 patients studied. One case of gynecomastia has been reported (personal communication).
> T1/2= 105 min.   Oral= 25-50%   Peak= 3-6 hours
> LRC= L2

ATENOLOL   **AAP**: Compatible
> **Trade:**   Tenoretic, Tenormin
> **Can/Aus/UK:**   Apo-Atenolol, Tenormin, Anselol, Noten, Tenlol, Tensig, Antipress
> ***Specifics:***   Atenolol is a second line choice beta-blocker, although it has been used in many breastfeeding women.   Metoprolol or propranolol should be considered first line.
> T1/2= 6.1 hours   Oral= 50-60%   Peak= 2-4 hours
> LRC= L3

BENAZEPRIL HCL   **AAP**: Not Reviewed
> **Trade:**   Lotensin
> **Can/Aus/UK:**
> ***Specifics:***   May be suitable, but studies are incomplete. Poor oral bioavailability. Captopril may be preferred.
> T1/2= 10-11 hours   Oral= 37%   Peak= 0.5 - 1 hr.
> LRC= L3
> > L4 if used in neonatal period

CAPTOPRIL   **AAP**: Compatible
> **Trade:**   Capoten
> **Can/Aus/UK:**   Capoten, Apo-Capto, Novo-Captopril, Acenorm, Capoten, Enzace, Acepril
> ***Specifics:***   Milk levels are very low (4.7 μg/Liter of milk). No adverse effect in 12 infants studied.   Avoid in early neonatal periods, infants may be excessively sensitive.
> T1/2= 2.2 hours   Oral= 60-75%   Peak= 1 hr.
> LRC= L3 if used after 30 days
> > L4 if used early postpartum

ENALAPRIL MALEATE   AAP: Compatible
   Trade: Vasotec
Can/Aus/UK: Vasotec, Amprace, Renitec, Innovace
Specifics: Studies show levels are quite low, but they were not done at steady state.   Captopril or benazepril may be preferred.   Avoid in early neonatal periods, infants may be excessively sensitive.
T1/2= 35 hours(metabolite) Oral= 60%   Peak= 0.5-1.5 hours
LRC= L2
      L4 if used early postpartum

FUROSEMIDE   AAP: Not Reviewed
   Trade: Lasix
Can/Aus/UK: Apo-Furosemide, Novo-Semide, Lasix, Frusemide, Uremide, Frusid
Specifics: Furosemide levels in milk are unreported but are believed to be low.   Oral bioavailability of furosemide in neonates is extremely poor.
T1/2= 92 minutes   Oral= 60-70%   Peak= 1-2 hours
LRC= L3

HYDROCHLOROTHIAZIDE   AAP: Compatible
   Trade: Hydrodiuril, Esidrix, Oretic
Can/Aus/UK: Amizide, Apo-Hydro, Direma, Diuchlor H, Dyazide, Esidrex, Hydrodiuril, Modizide, Novo-Hydrazide
Specifics: In one study of a mother receiving a 50 mg dose each morning, milk levels were almost 25% of maternal plasma levels.   The dose ingested (assuming milk intake of 600 ml)   would be approximately 50 µg/day, a clinically insignificant amount.   The concentration of HCTZ in the infant's serum was undetectable(< 20 ng/ml).
T1/2= 5.6-14 hours   Oral= 72%   Peak= 2 hours
LRC= L2

HYDRALAZINE   AAP: Compatible
   Trade: Apresoline
Can/Aus/UK: Apresoline, Novo-Hylazin, Apo-Hydralazine, Alphapress
Specifics: Milk levels are small and the amount ingested by infant is generally subclinical.   Good choice for pre-eclampsia, gestational and postpartum hypertension.
T1/2= 1.5-8 hours   Oral= 30-50%   Peak= 2 hours
LRC= L2

LABETALOL   AAP: Compatible
   Trade: Trandate, Normodyne
Can/Aus/UK: Trandate, Presolol, Labrocol
Specifics: In one study of 3 women receiving   600 mg, 600mg, or 1200

112

mg/day, the peak concentration of labetalol in breastmilk was 129, 223, and 662µg/L respectively. In only one infant were measurable plasma levels found, 18 µg/L following a maternal dose of 600 mg. Therefore, only small amounts are secreted into human milk (0.004% of maternal dose).

T1/2= 6-8 hours   Oral= 30-40%   Peak= 1-2 hours(oral)
LRC= L2

METOPROLOL   AAP: Compatible
Trade: Toprol XL, Lopressor
Can/Aus/UK: Apo-Metoprolol, Betaloc, Lopressor, Novo-Metoprol, Minax, Betaloc
Specifics: First line choice of beta-blocker for breastfeeding women. Milk levels are minimal. Side effects in infant are minimal.
T1/2= 3-7 hours   Oral= 40-50%   Peak= 2.5-3 hours
LRC= L3

NIFEDIPINE   AAP: Compatible
Trade: Adalat, Procardia
Can/Aus/UK: Adalat, Apo-Nifed, Novo-Nifedin, Nu-Nifed, Nifecard, Nyefax, Nefensar XL
Specifics: Milk levels of this calcium channel blocker are quite low. Its use in angina is not preferred.
T1/2= 1.8-7 hours   Oral= 50%   Peak= 45 min-4 hours
LRC= L2

VERAPAMIL   AAP: Compatible
Trade: Calan, Isoptin, Covera-HS
Can/Aus/UK: Apo-Verap, Isoptin, Novo-Veramil, Anpec, Cordilox, Veracaps SR, Berkatens, Univer
Specifics: Verapamil levels in milk are generally quite low, and side effects have not been noted in breastfeeding infants. Verapamil may also be used in panic and manic attacks. But because it reduces uterine contractility, discontinue prior to delivery.
T1/2= 3-7 hours   Oral= 90%   Peak= 1-2.2 hours
LRC= L2

NIMODIPINE   AAP: Not Reviewed
Trade: Nimotop
Can/Aus/UK: Nimotop
Specifics: Breastmilk levels are reported to be very low in at least several studies. No untoward effects were noted in the infants.
T1/2= 9 hours   Oral= 13%   Peak= 1 hour
LRC= L2

Clinical Tips:

Therapy of hypertension in younger patients generally starts with a beta-blocker or ACE inhibitor.   Of the beta-blocker family, metoprolol or labetalol are very cardioselective, and are preferred choices in breastfeeding patients.   Propranolol is another good choice, but its lack of beta receptor specificity is a problem (particularly asthmatics). Atenolol can and has been often used, but at least one case of bradycardia and hypotension has been reported.   This can occur with any beta-blocker.   When using beta-blockers be observant for bradycardia, hypotension, and apnea although, these are rare with the above agents.   The diuretics have been used extensively in breastfeeding women without problem.   Several members of the calcium channel blocker family have been studied.   Verapamil, nifedipine and nimodipine produce subclinical milk levels and appear relatively safe to use.   Of the ACE inhibitor family, captopril, nimodipine, and enalapril are transferred to milk in very low levels.   Nevertheless, neonates are very sensitive to ACE inhibitors, so be cautious of their use the first month postpartum.   Hydralazine has been used extensively early postpartum without problem in breastfed infants.   Because breastmilk production is dependent on blood supply and pressure, be aware that a drastic reduction in blood pressure may reduce the supply of milk.

Suggested Reading:

1. Lewis CE. Characteristics and treatment of hypertension in women: a review of the literature. Am J Med Sci. 1996 Apr;311(4):193-9. Review.
2. Kaplan NM. Treatment of hypertension: insights from the JNC-VI report. Am Fam Physician. 1998 Oct 15;58(6):1323-30. Review.
3. Hennekens CH. Lessons from hypertension trials. Am J Med. 1998 Jun 22;104(6A):50S-53S. Review.
4. Krieger JE. New contributions to clinical hypertension from molecular biology. Curr Opin Cardiol. 1998 Sep;13(5):312-6. Review.
5. Guidelines for Women's Health Care Second Edition, The American College of OB/Gyn.
6. 2002 Compenduium of Selected Publications The American College of OB/Gyn Women's Health Care Physicians, 2002.

Hyperthyroidism

Principles of Therapy:
Hyperthyroidism, commonly called Graves' disease, is one of the most frequent thyroid disorders, and is characterized by elevated circulating thyroid hormone, exophthalmos, goiter, and pretibial myxedema. It is known that Graves' disease results from stimulation of the thyroid gland by circulating antibodies to the thyroid stimulating hormone (TSH) receptor, although the mechanism is not completely understood. Once stimulated, the gland creates and releases high levels of thyroid hormones (T4 and/or T3) which are responsible for the symptoms. Therapy of hyperthyroidism requires a complete understanding of the endocrinology of this syndrome and should not be taken lightly. Treatment involves use of antithyroid medications, beta-blockers for treatment of thyroid storm (thyrotoxicosis), and radioactive Iodine for destruction of the gland in some cases.

METHIMAZOLE   AAP: Compatible

Trade: Tapazole
Can/Aus/UK:
Specifics: In 5 studies of over 187 hyperthyroid breastfeeding women treated with methimazole with doses as high as 20 mg/day, no changes in thyroid function were noted in any infant. In most infants, methimazole was undetectable in the plasma.
T½= 6-13 hours   Oral= 80-95%   Peak= 1 hr.
LRC= L3

PROPRANOLOL   AAP: Compatible

Trade: Inderal
Can/Aus/UK: Detensol, Inderal, Novo-Pranol, Deralin, Cardinol
Specifics: Propranolol is an ideal beta-blocker for breastfeeding women. Numerous studies show minimal milk levels and minimal to no side effects in the infant.
T½= 3-5 hours   Oral= 30%   Peak= 60-90 min.
LRC= L3

PROPYLTHIOURACIL   AAP: Compatible

Trade: PTU
Can/Aus/UK: PTU
Specifics: Numerous studies show only subclinical transfer of PTU to the infant via milk. No change in infant thyroid function has been reported.

T½= 1-2 hours   Oral= 50-95%   Peak= 1-1.5 hours
LRC= L2

Clinical Tips:

Initial therapy is to control the peripheral symptoms of excess thyroid hormone, symptoms such as tachycardia, atrial fibrillation, tremor, loss of body weight, sweating, heat intolerance, and intestinal hyperactivity. Usually 30-60 mg daily of propranolol is sufficient, but doses as high as 480 mg/day have been used. Propranolol has been studied in breastfeeding women and in most cases produces no untoward effect on the infant, but watch for hypotension and hypoglycemia. As Iodine concentrates in milk (25 fold), it should be avoided if possible in breastfeeding mothers as iodine transfer to the infant could be significant, enough to suppress thyroid function in the neonate. To suppress maternal thyroid function, propylthiouracil (PTU) is usually the drug of choice in breastfeeding mothers as its milk levels are the least. Numerous studies have been done and no change in thyroid function in any infant has been reported. PTU levels in milk are very low. Recent studies of methimazole suggest it is a suitable alternative. In 5 studies of over 187 hyperthyroid breastfeeding women treated with methimazole with doses as high as 20 mg/day, no changes in thyroid function were noted in any infant. In most infants, methimazole was undetectable in the plasma. While PTU is a preferred choice due to its suppression of peripheral conversion of T4 to T3, methimazole is undoubtedly safe as well. Monitoring for thyroid function and leukocytopenia in the breastfed neonate, while not mandatory, may be prudent. Radioactive ablation of the gland with Iodine-131 is especially dangerous to a breastfed infant. High doses of radioactive Iodine-131 are known to transfer via milk to the infant, and while not enough to destroy an infant's thyroid, they could predispose the infant to thyroid carcinoma in later years. Further, almost 40% of the I-131 dose is reposited directly into breast tissue of lactating women. Some authors suggest this may increase the risk of breast cancer. Therefore, the U.S. Nuclear Regulatory Commission recommends that the mother discontinue breastfeeding permanently for this infant. We concur and further recommend that the mother discontinue breastfeeding for at least several weeks prior to undergoing radiotherapy ablation for maximum protection of infant and mother. The U.S. Nuclear Regulatory Commission recommendations for use of radioactive materials in breastfeeding women are in Appendix A.

Suggested Reading:

1.   Haddad G. Is it hyperthyroidism? You can't always tell from the clinical picture. Postgrad Med. 1998 Jul;104(1):42-4, 53-5, 59. Review.
2.   Gittoes NJ, et al. Hyperthyroidism. Current treatment guidelines. Drugs. 1998 Apr;55(4):543-53. Review.
3.   McDermott MT, et al. Central hyperthyroidism. Endocrinol Metab Clin North Am. 1998 Mar;27(1):187-203. Review.
4.   Lazarus JH. Hyperthyroidism. Lancet. 1997 Feb 1;349(9048):339-43. Review.
5.   Hashizume K, et al. Hyperthyroidism. Curr Ther Endocrinol Metab. 1997;6:71-6.

Review.

6. Tegler L, Lindstrom B. Antithyroid drugs in milk. Lancet 2:591,1980.

7. Azizi F. Effect of methimazole treatment of maternal thyrotoxicosis on thyroid function in breast-feeding infants. J. Pediatr. 128:855-58, 1996.

8. Lamberg BA, Ikonen E, et.al. Antithyroid treatment of maternal hyperthyroidism during lactation. Clin. Endocrinol. 21(1):81-7, 1984.

9. Rylance GW; Woods CG; Donnelly MC; Oliver JS; Alexander WD. Carbimazole and breastfeeding [letter]. Lancet 18;1(8538):928, 1987.

10. Azizi F, Khoshniat M, Bahrainian M, Hedayati M. Thyroid function and intellectual development of infants nursed by mothers taking methimazole. J Clin Endocrinol Metab. 85(9):3233-8, 2000.

Hypothyroidism

Principles of Therapy:

Primary hypothyroidism is probably an autoimmune disease usually occurring as a sequel to Hashimoto's thyroiditis. While it can occur at any age, those at highest risk are the elderly and postmenopausal patients. Ultimately, hypothyroidism commonly results in a shrunken fibrotic gland with little function. Secondary hypothyroidism occurs when there is a failure of the hypothalamic-pituitary axis, leading to reduced levels of circulating Thyroid Stimulating Hormone (TSH). The treatment of hypothyroidism is generally replacement of the thyroid hormone (T4) and rarely T3. It is important to remember that it requires up to 6 weeks of therapy before steady-state levels of thyroxine are attained. In addition, serum TSH levels in hypothyroid patients reach their nadir within 6 weeks of beginning treatment. Therefore, thyroid function tests after 6 weeks are quite reliable in predicting if exogenous levothyroxine therapy is adequate. The nuances in discerning hypothyroid states are enormous and careful laboratory and/or clinical study of the patient by accomplished clinicians or an endocrinologist is important.

LEVOTHYROXINE   AAP: Not Reviewed

Trade: Synthroid, Levothroid, Thyroid, Levo-T, Levoxyl
Can/Aus/UK: Eltroxin, Synthroid, Thyroxine, Oroxine, Eltroxin
Specifics: Levels in breastmilk are exceptionally low (< 4 ng/mL), and will not protect a hypothyroid neonate.
$T\frac{1}{2}$= 6-7 days.   Oral= 50-80%   Peak= 2-4 hours
LRC= L1

LIOTHYRONINE   AAP: Not Reviewed

Trade: Cytomel
Can/Aus/UK: Cytomel, Tertroxin
Specifics: Milk levels are unreported, but are believed very low.
$T\frac{1}{2}$= 25 hours   Oral= 95 %   Peak= 1-2 hours
LRC= L2

Clinical Tips:

Treatment of hypothyroid disorders is generally initiated with synthetic levothyroxine sodium. Synthetic forms of thyroxine are more stable, are more standardized (potency), and are better absorbed in the GI tract (60-80% bioavailable). Thyroxine's long half-life of 6 days permits single-day dosing regimens with minimal day-to-day variability. Liothyronine (T3), due to a short 1 day half-life, is generally restricted to use in primary hypothyroidism in patients with thyroid cancer undergoing T4 withdrawal for thyroid scanning or ablation.

The transfer of levothyroxine into milk is extremely low. The amount of thyroid replacement varies during pregnancy and the post-partum period. Hormonal levels should be re-evaluated at the post-partum visit in patients with known hypothyroidism. Additionally, it is estimated that 5 to 10 % of women have evidence of some transient post-partum thyroid dysfunction that typically occurs after the common 6 week post-partum follow-up visit. It is well known that maternal hypothyroidism may be associated with low milk production, and this should be investigated in patients with extremely low milk supply.

Suggested Reading:

1. Weetman AP. Hypothyroidism: screening and subclinical disease. BMJ. 1997 Apr 19;314(7088):1175-8. Review.
2. Lindsay RS, et al. Hypothyroidism. Lancet. 1997 Feb 8;349(9049):413-7. Review.
3. Arem R, et al. Subclinical hypothyroidism: epidemiology, diagnosis, and significance. Adv Intern Med. 1996;41:213-50. Review.
4. Mizuta H, Amino N, Ichihara K et al: Thyroid hormones in human milk and their influence on thyroid function of breast-fed babies. Pediatr Res 17:468-471, 1983.
5. Oberkotter LV, Hahn HB. Thyroid function and human breast milk. Am .J Dis Child. 137:1131, 1983
6. Sack J. et. Al. Thyroxine concentration in human milk. J Clin Endocrinol Metab 45:171-3, 1977.
7. Anderson PO. Drugs and breast feeding – a review. Drug Intell Clin Pharm 11:208, 1977.
8. Varma SK, et.al. Thyroxine, triiodothyronine, and reverse triiodothyronine concentrations in human milk. J. Pediatr. 93:803-6, 1978.

Infectious Disease – Acute Sinusitis

Principles of Therapy:

The clinical manifestations of acute sinusitis vary greatly, depending on the duration of infection (acute or chronic), and the age of the patient. Acute sinusitis is defined as inflammation of the sinuses with symptoms that have persisted for less than 4 weeks. Subacute sinusitis is defined as inflammation of the sinuses with symptoms lasting 1-3 months. Chronic sinusitis is associated with inflammatory symptoms lasting more than 3 months. Sinusitis generally develops because of impaired clearance of secretions resulting from obstruction of the sinus ostia by infection, inflammation or anatomic abnormalities, or an increased viscosity of sinus secretions. Due to impaired drainage, an overgrowth of pathogenic bacteria results. Symptoms of infectious or acute sinusitis are difficult to distinguish from the symptoms of the common cold or allergic rhinitis. Because acute sinusitis often occurs soon after or in conjunction with allergic vasomotor rhinitis, it is generally believed that allergic rhinitis may in some cases predispose to acute infectious sinusitis. In adults, purulent postnasal discharge and facial pain over the affected sinus that worsens with movement are the typical symptoms. Fever occurs in fewer than 50% of cases. Jaw pain with chewing, nasal congestion and pressure, and a history of a recent upper respiratory tract infection are other manifestations. Symptoms of subacute or chronic infections are subtle and difficult to diagnose. Fever is usually absent. Fatigue, malaise, and irritability are most common. Chronic sinusitis may mimic asthma, allergic rhinitis, or chronic inflammatory bronchitis. Approximately 40% of chronic sinusitis patients have dental problems. Bacterial etiologies: Strep. Pneumonia 40%, H. influenzae 30%, M.Catarrhalis 7%, anaerobes 8%, viruses 15%, and Staph. Aureus 4%.

AMOXICILLIN + CLAVULANATE   AAP: Compatible

Trade: Larotid, Amoxil
Can/Aus/UK: Amoxil, Apo-Amoxi, Novamoxin, Alphamox, Moxacin, Cilamox, Betamox
Specifics: Amoxicillin levels in milk are low and average 0.9 mg/Liter of milk or lower. Current studies show amoxicillin by itself is no more effective than placebo in infectious sinusitis.
T½= 1.7 hours   Oral= 89%   Peak= 1.5 hours
LRC= L1

AZITHROMYCIN   AAP: Not Reviewed

Trade: Zithromax
Can/Aus/UK: Zithromax
Specifics: In one study of a patient who received 1 gm initially, followed by two 500mg doses at 24 hr intervals, the concentration of azithromycin in breastmilk varied from 0.64 mg/L (initially) to 2.8 mg/L on day 3. The predicted dose of azithromycin received by the infant would be approximately 0.482 mg/day.
T½= 48-68 hours   Oral= 37%   Peak= 3-4 hours
LRC= L2

CEFPROZIL   AAP: Compatible

Trade: Cefzil
Can/Aus/UK:
Specifics: Following an oral dose of 1000 mg, the breastmilk concentrations were 0.7, 2.5, and 3.4 mg/L at 2, 4, and 6 hours post-dose respectively. The peak milk concentration occurred at 6 hours, and was lower thereafter.
T½= 78 minutes   Oral= Complete   Peak= 1.5 hours
LRC= L1

CEFPODOXIME   AAP: Not Reviewed

Trade: Vantin
Can/Aus/UK: Orelox
Specifics: In a study of 3 lactating women, levels of cefpodoxime in human milk were 0%, 2%, and 6% of maternal serum levels at 4 hours following a 200 mg oral dose. At 6 hours post-dosing, levels were 0%, 9%, and 16% of concomitant maternal serum levels.
T½= 2.09-2.84 hours   Oral= 50%   Peak= 2-3 hours
LRC= L2

CEFUROXIME   AAP: Not Reviewed

Trade: Ceftin, Zinacef, Kefurox
Can/Aus/UK:
Specifics: Milk levels are believed to be low, but are unreported.
T½= 1.4 hours   Oral= 30-50%   Peak= N/A
LRC= L2

CLARITHROMYCIN
AAP: Not Reviewed

Trade: Biaxin
Can/Aus/UK: Biaxin, Klacid
Specifics: Levels in milk are unknown, but most macrolide antibiotics are cleared for use in breastfeeding mothers.
T½= 5-7 hours   Oral= 50%   Peak= 1.7 hours
LRC= L2

CO-TRIMOXAZOLE
AAP: Compatible

Trade: TMP-SMZ, Bactrim, CoTrim, Septra
Can/Aus/UK: Novo-Trimel, Septrin, Bactrim, Respax, Trimogal
Specifics: Mixture of trimethoprim and sulfamethoxazole. Trimethoprim levels vary from 1.2-5.5 mg/liter of milk.

LEVOFLOXACIN
AAP: Not Reviewed

Trade: Levaquin, Quixin
Can/Aus/UK: Levaquin
Specifics: Levofloxacin is a pur (S) enantiomer of the racemic ofloxacin. Its kinetics and milk levels should be the same as ofloxacin. See ofloxacin below..
T½= 6-8 hours   Oral= 99 %   Peak= 1-1.8 hours
LRC= L3

OFLOXACIN
AAP: Not Reviewed

Trade: Floxin
Can/Aus/UK: Floxin, Ocuflox, Tarivid
Specifics: In one study in lactating women who received 400 mg oral doses twice daily, drug concentrations in breastmilk averaged 0.05-2.41 mg/L in milk (24 hours and 2 hours post-dose respectively). Milk levels are much lower than ciprofloxacin levels.
T½= 5-7 hours   Oral= 98 %   Peak= 0.5-2 hours
LRC= L3

TROVAFLOXACIN MESYLATE
AAP: Not Reviewed

Trade: Trovan, Alatrofloxacin
Can/Aus/UK:
Specifics: Reported milk levels are very low and averaged 0.8 mg/Liter of milk. Recent data suggest this product may be hepatotoxic and caution is recommended.
T½= 12.2 hours   Oral= 88%   Peak= 1-2 hours
LRC= L4

Clinical Tips:

The goals of treatment are to eradicate the offending organism, clear sinuses, provide symptomatic relief and prevent intracranial complications. The choice of antibiotic varies due to age of patients. In adults, empiric therapy should be initially directed against *H. influenza* and *Strep. Pneumoniae*. While a 10-14 day course of amoxicillin may be tried, current studies show most strains are resistant and response is no better than placebo. First choice is probably amoxicillin + clavulanic acid (500/125 mg TID or 875/125 mg BID PO x 10 days), or cefuroxime axetil (250 mg BID x 10 days), or TMP-SMX (160/800 mg q 12 hours). Alternative treatments include cefprozil or cefpodoxime. In penicillin-allergic patients, clarithromycin (500mg po BID x 10 days) or azithromycin (250 mg daily for 5 days) may be used. All of the above chemotherapeutic agents have been studied in breastfeeding mothers and levels in milk are low. While the incidence of resistance is growing, the use of fluoroquinolone antibiotics is increasing as well. Although ciprofloxacin is useful, it may produce higher milk levels(40%) than other fluoroquinolones, and it should be used cautiously in breastfeeding mothers. Pseudomembranous colitis has been reported in one infant. In patients needing fluoroquinolones, ofloxacin(400 mg q 12 hours x 10 days) or levofloxacin would be preferred due to lower levels in milk. The only consequence of using the fluoroquinolones is the possibility of overgrowth of *C. Difficle* which at these doses via milk is low.

Suggested Reading:

1.   Chow A.W. Infections of the Sinuses and Parameningeal Structures In: Infectious Diseases. Gorbach S.L. eds. W.B. Saunders, Philadephia, 1998.
2.   Gilbert DN, Moellering RC, Sande MA. The Sandford guide to antimicrobial therapy 1998.
3.   Bone R.C. The pathogenesis of sepsis. Ann Intern Med 115:457-469, 1991.

Infectious Disease – Candida Albicans

Principles of Therapy:

Candidiasis is the most common mucosal and invasive fungal infection in humans, and Candida albicans is the most common species. Fungal infections, particularly candida, have increased in incidence due to the extensive use of antibiotics. Other Candida species include: C. glabrata, C. tropicalis, C. parapisilosis, and C. krusei. C. albicans is a normal flora and can be cultured from the mouth, feces, and vagina in most normal humans. The major risk factors for invasive candidiasis include: pregnancy, diabetes, recent surgery, use of broad spectrum antibiotics, corticosteroid therapy, neutropenia and impaired cell-mediated immunity (HIV infection). Cutaneous candidiasis is most commonly associated with areas of increased moisture, such as intertriginous and inguinal areas, the vulva, and in breastfeeding mothers, the nipple and areola. Breast infections with candida may be excruciatingly painful for the mother despite a paucity of clinical finding on inspection of the breast. Mucosal candidiasis can develop in the oropharynx, esophagus, gastrointestinal tract, vaginal mucosa, and urinary tract. Diagnosis of vulvovaginal Candidiasis (VVC) is made either by signs and symptoms or on the basis of inspection of vaginal discharge using 10% KOH prepared slides under the microscope evaluating for budding hyphae. Diagnosis of breast infection is primarily based on signs, symptoms and clinical suspicion. Cultures for yeast are of little clinical use as culture techniques are limited and presence of the organism does not indicate clinical infection. The therapy of candidiasis largely depends on the location and severity of the infection. Topical candidiasis therapy includes reduction of moisture and the use of topical antifungals such as nystatin, miconazole, butoconazole, tioconazole, terconazole or clotrimazole. Multiple intravaginal versions of these agents are available over the counter for treatment of VVC. Recommended systemic therapy includes the use of fluconazole. Itraconazole or ketoconazole are less desirable alternatives. Hepatotoxicity related to ketoconazole is rare but more common than with fluconazole. Drug–drug interactions are an important consideration to remember with the use of systemic medications. Some studies suggest that nystatin resistance has increased and almost 45% of candida strains are resistant to Nystatin in certain populations. A study of oral candida in an otherwise healthy population found 88% of patients to be culture positive for C. albicans with testing revealing that all strains were susceptible to fluconazole. Epidemiologic information on candidemia from 1998 to 2001 done in Iowa found only 3% of Candida species to be resistant to fluconazole. In breastfeeding mothers, fluconazole is probably preferred as milk levels are known to be low and its toxicity in infants is minimal. Further, fluconazole is cleared for use in infants 6 months and older. Vulvovaginal Candidiasis (VVC) is quite common with 75% of women experiencing at least one infection. Symptoms may include vaginal dischange, vulvar itching and irritation and dysparunia.

BUTOCONAZOLE   **AAP**: Not Reviewed
Trade: Femstat, Mycelex
Can/Aus/UK:
Specifics: Serum levels are measurable 2 to 8 hours after vaginal administration, and peak at 24 hours. Systemic absorption from vagina is estimated to be about 5%. Useful primarily for VVC as a 2% cream, 5 gms intravaginaly for 3 days.
T1/2= 21 hours   Oral= 5.5% vaginal   Peak= 24 hours
LRC= L3

CLOTRIMAZOLE   **AAP**: Not Reviewed
Trade: Gyne-Lotrimin, Mycelex, Lotrimin, Femcare
Can/Aus/UK: Canesten, Clotrimaderm, Myclo, Clonea, Hiderm
Specifics: Systemic absorption following intravaginal use is minimal (< 3-10%). Useful either for nipple infections (for mother and infant) or for VVC. Various treatment regimes are available.
T1/2= 3.5-5 hours   Oral= Poor   Peak= 3 hours (oral)
LRC= L1

FLUCONAZOLE   **AAP**: Not Reviewed
Trade: Diflucan
Can/Aus/UK: Diflucan
Specifics: Published milk levels are quite low and are not sufficient to treat the breastfed infant. Peak levels of fluconazole are 2.93 mg/Liter of milk or less than 5% of the recommended pediatric dose. Used in treatment of either systemic infection, breast infection VVC at different doses.
T1/2= 30 hours   Oral= >90%   Peak= 1-2 hours
LRC= L2

GENTIAN VIOLET   **AAP**: Not Reviewed
Trade: Crystal Violet, Methylrosaniline Chloride, Gentian Violet
Can/Aus/UK:
Specifics: Gentian violet kills candida on contact and is becoming more popular for oral thrush because of resistance to nystatin. Paint infants' mouth (including mothers' nipple and areola) once daily for no more than 3-7 days. Useful predominately for nipple candidiasis
T1/2= N/A   Oral= N/A   Peak= N/A
LRC= L3

KETOCONAZOLE   AAP: Not Reviewed
Trade: Nizoral
Can/Aus/UK: Nizoral
Specifics: Ketoconazole levels in milk have not been determined, but it would likely be poorly bioavailable in the GI tract of an infant due to the presence of milk and low acidity.
T1/2= 2-8 hours   Oral= Variable (75%)   Peak= 1-2 hours
LRC= L2

MICONAZOLE   AAP: Not Reviewed
Trade: Monistat-Derm, Monistat Vaginal Cream 2%
Can/Aus/UK: Micatin, Monistat, Daktarin, Daktozin, Fungo
Specifics: Good azole topical antifungal. This is an ideal topical choice for the nipple as the oral bioavailability is minimal (< 25%).   Useful either for nipple infections (for mother and infant) or for VVC. Various treatment regimes are available
T1/2= 20-25 hours   Oral= 25-30%   Peak= Immediate(IV)
LRC= L2

NYSTATIN   AAP: Not Reviewed
Trade: Mycostatin, Nilstat
Can/Aus/UK: Mycostatin, Nadostine, Nilstat, Candistatin, Nystan
Specifics: Oral bioavailability is nil.   While extremely safe, it is poorly efficacious.
T1/2= N/A   Oral= Poor   Peak= N/A
LRC= L1

TIOCONAZOLE   AAP: Not Reviewed
Trade:
Can/Aus/UK:
Specifics: Useful primarily for VVC. Recommended dosage 6.5% ointment, 5 gms given as single intravaginal application. Topical absorption is minimal. Plasma levels minimal.   Transcutaneous absorption is only 2.9%; vaginal absorption is negligible.
T1/2= N/A   Oral= Nil   Peak= 12 hours
LRC= L3

TERCONAZOLE   **AAP**: Not Reviewed

Trade: Terazol
Can/Aus/UK: Terazol
Specifics: Terconazole is a triazole antifungal agent for the treatment of vulvovaginal candidiasis.   Useful primarily for VVC.   Various treatment regimes are available.   Approximately 5% to 16% of an intravaginal dose is absorbed systemically.
T1/2= 6-12 hours   Oral= 5-16% vag.   Peak= 6.6 hours
LRC= L3

Clinical Tips:

Because thrush is so common in infants and breastfeeding mothers, it is quite common for candida to pass back and forth repeatedly from infant to mother. Therefore, it is often recommended that both mother and infant be treated simultaneously.   Candida in the breastfeeding mother commonly occurs on the nipple or areola.   Cutaneous candidiasis is best treated with topical nystatin, miconazole, clotrimazole, or gentian violet.   Because nystatin is poorly effective, miconazole or clotrimazole are more effective choices today.   For candida of the nipple, miconazole is ideal (due to poor bioavailability in the infant), but clotrimazole is also effective. Apply small amounts after breastfeeding four to eight times daily.   Due to the poor oral bioavailability there is no need to wipe any remaining cream from the nipple prior to feeding which could further contribute to nipple trauma. Gentian violet is increasing in popularity for thrush and nipple candida as candida strains become more resistant to therapy.   Weak aqueous solutions 0.5-1% can be applied directly to the nipple and areola, or applied in the mouth of the infant once daily for no more than 3-7 days. Gentian violet can irritate mucus membranes and care should be exercised that it is not used for more than one week at any time.   In some breastfeeding patients, candida is believed to invade ductal tissues of the breast producing a deep shooting pain into the axilla or chest wall and persisting throughout the feeding and frequently lasting after the feeding is completed. This should be considered systemic candidiasis and responds best to oral fluconazole (200-400 mg STAT, followed by 100-200 mg daily for 14-21 days). Fluconazole levels in breastmilk are quite low and are not enough to be clinically effective in the infant, hence the infant may require additional therapy including fluconazole, nystatin, or gentian violet. With candidial breast infections, it is generally recommended that both mother and infant are treated simultaneously, even in situations where only one is symptomatic.   Plastic-backed breastpads retain moisture and warmth from the body providing an ideal environment for yeast. Their use should be avoided.   Other hygienic maneuvers should also be taken such as meticulous washing / boiling of any items in contact with mothers affected nipples or baby's mouth. Vulvovaginal Candidiasis (VVC) in the breastfeeding patient can be treated with topical miconazole or clotrimazole creams or one 150 mg tablet (PO) of fluconazole. Recurrent VVC is often treated by 150mgs oral fluconazole with repeat dosing given 72 hours later. C. glabrata may be causative in patients with recurrent VVC. The single oral dose of fluconazole is not sufficient for treating systemic candidiasis and is not effective in ductal candidiasis in breastfeeding patients

Suggested Reading:

1. McCullough MJ, et al. Candida albicans: a review of its history, taxonomy, epidemiology, virulence attributes, and methods of strain differentiation. Int J Oral Maxillofac Surg. 1996 Apr;25(2):136-44. Review.
2. Corner BE, et al. Candida pathogenesis: unraveling the threads of infection. Curr Biol. 1997 Nov 1;7(11):R691-4. Review.
3. Pfaller MA. Epidemiology of candidiasis. J Hosp Infect. 1995 Jun;30 Suppl:329-38. Review.
4. Faergemann, J. Pharmacokietics of fluconazole in skin and nails. J. Amer. Acad. Dermatol. 40(6):S14-20, 1999.

Infectious Disease - Chlamydia

Principles of Therapy:

Infection with *C. trachomatis* is one of the most common genitourinary tract infections occurring in adolescents and women in their 20's in the USA. Chlamydia trachomatis accounts for at least 50% of reported cases of non-gonococcal urethritis. Most women are asymptomatic, although vaginal discharge, dysuria, urinary frequency, pelvic pain and dyspareunia may occur. Cervicitis with the characteristic yellow, mucopurulent secretion is present. In women, gram stains of mucopurulent discharge often shows many leukocytes but no gonococci. Complications of C. trachomatis are numerous and include: bartholinitis, perihepatitis, chlamydial salpingitis, Reiter's syndrome, chlamydial ophthalmia neonatorum, chronic pelvic pain, ectopic pregnancy, infertility etc.

AZITHROMYCIN   AAP: Not Reviewed
Trade: Zithromax
Can/Aus/UK: Zithromax
Specifics: Azithromycin levels in milk are very low.
T1/2= 48-68 hours   Oral= 37%   Peak= 3-4 hours
LRC= L2

CIPROFLOXACIN   AAP: Compatible
Trade: Cipro
Can/Aus/UK: Cipro, Ciloxan, Ciproxin
Specifics: Milk levels of ciprofloxacin vary enormously according to study, but probably vary according to dose from 1-4 mg/Liter of milk following oral use. Only one case of C. Difficile overgrowth has been reported. Ophthalmic use of ciprofloxacin produces minimal plasma levels and the amount entering milk would be minimal.
T1/2= 4.1 hours   Oral= 50-85%   Peak= 0.5-2.3 hours
LRC= L4

DOXYCYCLINE   AAP: Not Reviewed
Trade: Doxychel, Vibramycin
Can/Aus/UK: Apo-Doxy, Doxycin, Vibramycin, Vibra-Tabs, Doryx, Doxylin, Doxylar
Specifics: Milk levels are low (< 0.77 mg/L). Oral bioavailability is reduced (20%) in milk but not eliminated. Limited use is unlikely to produce side effects.
T1/2= 15-25 hours   Oral= 90-100%   Peak= 1.5-4 hours
LRC= L3
          L4 if used chronically

ERYTHROMYCIN   AAP: Compatible
Trade: E-Mycin, Ery-tab, Eryc, Ilosone
Can/Aus/UK: E-Mycin, Eryc, Erythromid, Novo-Rythro, PCE, Ilotyc, EMU-V, Ilosone, EES, E-Mycin, Erythrocin, Ceplac, Erycen
Specifics: Reported milk levels are less than 1.5 mg/Liter, generally considered subclinical.
T1/2= 1.5-2 hours   Oral= Variable   Peak= 2-4 hours
LRC= L1

OFLOXACIN   AAP: Not Reviewed
Trade: Floxin
Can/Aus/UK: Floxin, Ocuflox, Tarivid
Specifics: In one study in lactating women who received 400 mg oral doses twice daily, drug concentrations in breastmilk averaged 0.05-2.41 mg/L in milk (24 hours and 2 hours post-dose respectively). Milk levels are much lower than ciprofloxacin levels.
T1/2= 5-7 hours   Oral= 98 %   Peak= 0.5-2 hours
LRC= L3

TROVAFLOXACIN MESYLATE   AAP: Not Reviewed
Trade: Trovan, Alatrofloxacin
Can/Aus/UK:
Specifics: Reported milk levels are very low and averaged 0.8 mg/Liter of milk. Recent data suggest this product may be hepatotoxic and caution is recommended.
T1/2= 12.2 hours   Oral= 88%   Peak= 1-2 hours
LRC= L4

Clinical Tips:

Recommended treatment includes either Azithromycin or Doxycycline. Azithromycin as a single dose of 1 gm orally is preferred due to its ease of compliance and its documented efficacy. Doxycycline 100mgs twice daily for 7 days may also be used though Azithromycin is a better choice for breastfeeding mothers. The alternative treatment is erythromycin base 500 mg four times daily or Erthromycin ethylsuccinate (EES) 800mgs four times daily for 7 days. Erythromycin formulations are less efficacious and are limited by nausea and vomiting as frequent side effects. Ofloxacin (300 mg PO BID for 7 days) has similar efficacy as either azithromycin or doxycycline but is more expensive and has no advantage over the azithromycin. Patients should be instructed to refrain from sexual intercourse for 7 days after treatment and partners should be referred for treatment.

Suggested Reading:

1. Marrazzo JM, et al. New approaches to the diagnosis, treatment, and prevention of chlamydial infection. Curr Clin Top Infect Dis. 1998;18:37-59. Review.
2. Schubiner H, et al. Chlamydia trachomatis infections in women. Curr Probl Dermatol. 1996;24:25-33. Review.
3. Heath CB, et al. Chlamydia trachomatis infection update. Am Fam Physician. 1995 Oct;52(5):1455-62. Review.
4. MMWR 1998 Guidelines for Teatment of Sexually Transmitted Disease January 23, 1998 Vol/47No.RR-1 Recommendations and Reports.
5. 2002 Compenduium of Selected Publications The American College of OB/Gyn Women's Health Care Physicians, 2002.

Infectious Disease - Giardiasis

Principles of Therapy:
Giardiasis is an infection of the small intestine caused by Giardia lamblia, a flagellated protozoan. The infection is found worldwide, especially in children where sanitation conditions are poor.   Risks are higher for patients with HIV, gastrectomies, lower gastric acidity and immunodeficiencies.   Symptoms in adults may be acute or chronic, usually mild, and consist of nausea, flatulence, epigastric pain, abdominal cramps, malodorous stools and diarrhea. Acute diarrhea due to giardiasis can be differentiated from other intestinal infections by the lack of blood or mucous in the stools,   presence of upper abdominal cramping, distention and malodorous stools.

FURAZOLIDONE   AAP: Not Reviewed

Trade: Furoxone
Can/Aus/UK:
Specifics: Poor oral bioavailability would limit absorption by infant. Milk levels are unreported.
T½= N/A   Oral= < 5%   Peak= N/A
LRC= L3

METRONIDAZOLE   AAP: May be of concern

Trade: Flagyl, Metizol, Trikacide, Protostat
Can/Aus/UK: Apo-Metronidazole, Flagyl, NeoMetric, Novo-Nidazol, Metrozine, Rozex
Specifics: Milk levels are moderate to low. Metronidazole concentrations in milk vary widely from 9.9% to 13% of the maternal dose at doses of 0.6 g/d to 1.2 g/d. Milk levels are quite high following the 2 g Stat dose for a few hours, and a 12-24 hour interruption of nursing is suggested at this dose.   No untoward effects have been reported in breastfed infants in numerous studies.
T½= 8.5 hours   Oral= Complete   Peak= 2-4 hours
LRC= L2

Clinical Tips:
The treatment of adult giardiasis as recommended by the World Health Organization is metronidazole in a dose of 250 mg TID for 5 days.   In some cases furazolidone (100mg QID X 7 days) can be used.   Although metronidazole has been found to be mutagenic in rodents, it has been used for years in adult and pediatric patients without reported mutagenicity.   Metronidazole entry into breastmilk has been well studied and is moderate and dose dependent.   Metronidazole concentrations in milk vary widely from 9.9% to 13% of the maternal dose at doses of 0.6 g/d to 1.2 g/d.

Milk levels are quite high following the 2 g Stat dose for a few hours, and a 12-24 hour interruption of nursing is suggested at this dose. No untoward effects have been reported in breastfed infants in numerous studies.

Suggested Reading:
1. Farthing MJ. Giardiasis. Gastroenterol Clin North Am. 1996 Sep;25(3):493-515. Review.
2. Babb RR. Giardiasis. Taming this pervasive parasitic infection. Postgrad Med. 1995 Aug;98(2):155-8. Review.
3. Zaat JO, et al. A systematic review on the treatment of giardiasis. Trop Med Int Health. 1997 Jan;2(1):63-82. Review.

Infectious Disease - Gonorrhea

Principles of Therapy:

Gonorrhea is the acute infectious disease of the epithelium of the urethra, cervix, rectum, pharynx or eyes that may lead to bacteremia and metastatic complications. The causative organism is Neisseria gonorrhoeae and is identified in discharges as pairs or clumps of gram-negative diplococci. The disease is spread by sexual contact. Women are often asymptomatic carriers of the organisms for weeks or months and may only be identified by tracing sexual partners. In men, the incubation period is 2-14 days. Onset is marked by mild discomfort in the urethra, dysuria and purulent discharge. In women, symptoms usually begin 7-21 days after infection. Symptoms are generally mild and include dysuria, frequency and vaginal discharge. Often women may be asymptomatic until symptoms of pelvic inflammatory disease are present. Treatment of gonorrhea has become more complicated due to the high frequency of concurrent infection with *Chlamydia trachomatis* in some populations. Depending on the frequency of coinfection in the particular population, it may be more cost effective to treat for presumed coinfection with chlamydia than screen for the disease. An additional concern is the increasing resistance of *N. gonorrhoeae* to penicillins. *N. gonorrhea* resistance to fluoroquinolone antibiotics has also been sporadically reported though this is presently rare (< 0.05%) in the United States. There are numerous treatment regimens available and the clinician must choose according to sensitivity and allergies of patient, and sensitivity of the organism.

AZITHROMYCIN   AAP: Not Reviewed
   Trade: Zithromax
   Can/Aus/UK: Zithromax
   Specifics: Azithromycin levels in milk are very low.
   T1/2= 48-68 hours   Oral= 37%   Peak= 3-4 hours
   LRC= L2

CEFIXIME   AAP: Not Reviewed
   Trade: Suprax
   Can/Aus/UK:
   Specifics: Milk levels are low, often undetectable. Oral bioavailability is poor (< 30-50%).
   T1/2= 7 hours   Oral= 30-50%   Peak= 2-6 hours
   LRC= L2

CEFTRIAXONE   AAP: Not Reviewed
   Trade: Rocephin
   Can/Aus/UK: Rocephin
   Specifics: Small amounts are transferred into milk (3-4% of maternal serum level).
Following a 1 gm IM dose, breastmilk levels were approximately 0.5-0.7 mg/L between
4-8 hours. The estimated mean milk levels at steady state were 3-4 mg/L. Another
source indicates that following a 2 g/d dose and at steady state, approximately 4.4 % of
dose penetrates into milk. In this study, the maximum breastmilk concentration was 7.89
mg/L after prolonged therapy (7days). Using this data, the weight-adjusted relative
infant dose would only be 0.35% of the maternal dose. Poor oral absorption of
ceftriaxone would further limit systemic absorption by the infant.
   T½= 7.3 hours   Oral= Poor   Peak= 1 hour
   LRC= L2

DOXYCYCLINE   AAP: Not Reviewed
   Trade: Doxychel, Vibramycin
   Can/Aus/UK: Apo-Doxy, Doxycin, Vibramycin, Vibra-Tabs, Doryx,
   Doxylin, Doxylar
   Specifics: Milk levels are low (< 0.77 mg/L). Oral bioavailability is reduced
(20%) in milk but not eliminated. Limited use is unlikely to produce side
effects.
   T1/2= 15-25 hours   Oral= 90-100%   Peak= 1.5-4 hours
   LRC= L3
             L4 if used chronically

OFLOXACIN   AAP: Not Reviewed
   Trade: Floxin
   Can/Aus/UK: Floxin, Ocuflox, Tarivid
   Specifics: Milk levels are low (much lower than ciprofloxacin levels).
   T1/2= 5-7 hours   Oral= 98 %   Peak= 0.5-2 hours
   LRC= L3

Clinical Tips:

Recommended therapy for a breastfeeding woman is ceftriaxone 125 mg IM.
Treatment for possible chlamydia is also recommended with either doxycycline (100
mg BID for 7 days) or azithromycin (1 gm single dose).   Although the risks of
doxycycline are remote, azithromycin therapy may be a better choice in
breastfeeding patients.   Azithromycin levels in milk are very low.   The
fluoroquinolones are sometimes recommended for gonorrhea but are not ideal for
breastfeeding patients. However, a single dose of ciprofloxacin (500 mg), or
ofloxacin (400mg) can be substituted for ceftriaxone if needed, and would be very
unlikely to harm a breastfeeding infant. Cefixime 400mgs orally can also be

substituted for ceftriaxone IM. Cefixime has a slightly lower clinical cure rate of approximately 97% compared to the 99% or better cure rate with ceftriaxone. A 2 gram single oral dose of Azithromycin is an effective alternative treatment for both gonorrhea and chlamydia. Potential drawbacks to this method include cost and possible gastrointestinal side effects. As with treatment for Chlamydia, patients with gonorrhea should be instructed to refer their sexual partners for therapy and should refrain from intercourse until after treatment has been given.

Suggested Reading:

1.   Miller KE. Women's health. Sexually transmitted diseases. Prim Care. 1997 Mar;24(1):179-93. Review.
2.   Sherrard J. Modern diagnosis and management of gonorrhoea. Br J Hosp Med. 1996 Apr 3-16;55(7):394-8. Review.
3.   Lind I. Gonorrhoea. Curr Probl Dermatol. 1996;24:12-9. Review.
4.   MMWR 1998 Guidelines for Teatment of Sexually Transmitted Disease January 23, 1998 Vol/47No.RR-1 Recommendations and Reports.
5.   2002 Compenduium of Selected Publications The American College of OB/Gyn Women's Health Care Physicians, 2002.

Infectious Disease - Hepatitis A

Principles of Therapy:

Hepatitis A is a RNA viral infection. Approximately one-third of cases of acute hepatitis are caused by this infection. It may be transmitted by person to person contact, sexual contacts and by fecal-oral spread related to poor sanitation or poor hygiene techniques. Travel to endemic areas or epidemic outbreaks due to contaminated uncooked food or water may also be implicated in this infection. The incubation period may be from 15 to 50 days. Hepatitis A infection is usually a self limited infection with fewer than 20% of patients requiring hospitalization. Treatment is usually supportive consisting of intravenous hydration. No chronic carrier state exists and fatal outcomes related to this disease are rare (2/1,000). Perinatal transmission or transmission via breastfeeding have not been documented. Careful hygiene should be effective in preventing tranmission to the breastfed infant. Treatment options available to prevent hepatitis A include immune globulin and inactivated hepatitis A vaccination.

IMMUNE GLOBULIN (HUMAN)   **AAP**: Not Reviewed
    Trade: BayGam, IG, IGIM, Gamma Globulin, IgG
    Can/Aus/UK:
    Specifics: Immune globulin is > 85% effective in preventing hepatitis A when given prior to or within < 2 weeks after exposure to the virus. Duration of protection lasts only approximately 3 to 6 months.

HEPATITIS A VACCINATION, INACTIVATED   **AAP**: Not Reviewed
    Trade: Havrix, Vaqta
    Can/Aus/UK:
    Specifics: Inactivated hepatitis A vaccinations are between 94-100% effective. A two dose series is recommended.

Clinical Tips:

Good personal hygiene should be protective against spreading hepatitis A. Post-exposure prophylaxis is indicated for household and sexual contacts of those recently exposed to a person infected with hepatitis A unless the exposed person has been vaccinated at least 1 month prior. Hepatitis A immune globulin (IG) is a dose of 0.02ml/kg should be administered within <2 weeks of exposure. Breastfeeding women who are otherwise candidates for either immune globulin or vaccination should be given treatment. It is unclear if the potential exposure of a breastfed infant to an infected mother would warrant treatment of the infant providing meticulous hygiene and adequate sanitation exist. Breastfeeding should continue during hepatitis A infection and therapy.

Suggested Reading:

1. MMWR 1998 Guidelines for Teatment of Sexually Transmitted Disease January 23, 1998 Vol/47No.RR-1 Recommendations and Reports.
2. 2002 Compenduium of Selected Publications The American College of OB/Gyn Women's Health Care Physicians, 2002.
3. Merewood A, Philipp BL. Breastfeeding Condition and Diseases First Edition, Pharmasoft Publishing 2001.

Infectious Disease - Hepatitis B

Principles of Therapy:

Hepatitis B (HBV) is caused by a DNA virus. Three principal antigens exist which are useful for testing for infection: hepatitis B surface antigen (HbsAg), hepatitis B core antigen (HBcAg) and hepatitis B e antigen (HbeAg). Presence of HbeAg indicates higher probability of infectivty. Approximately 40-45% of hepatitis in the United States is related to hepatitis B. Hepatitis B is spread through sexual contacts and exposure to infected blood such as occurs with blood transfusion or shared needles with intravenous drug use. Acute HBV infection carries a mortality of about 1%. Chronic HBV infection occurs in 1-15% of cases and can lead to further transmission of the infection as well as chronic liver disease potentially leading to cirrhosis and hepatocellular carcinoma. Diagnosis of chronic HBV infection is made based on a persistently postive test for HbsAg. Perinatal transmission of hepatitis B without treatment ranges from 10 to 85% depending on timing of infection and e antigen status. Those with a positive e antigen and infection in the third trimester of pregnancy are at greatest risk. Transmission via breastfeeding and/or close postnatal contact has also been reported. Chronic HBV infection occurs in 90% of infected newborns who are at especially high risk for chronic liver disease. Immune globulin and vaccination are recommended for all potentially exposed infants. No adequate treatment is available for hepatitis B infection once acute infection occurs. Care again focuses on supportive measures. Chronic HBV infection has been treated with interferon alpha-2b with approximately 25-40% efficacy. Options available to prevent hepatitis B infection include immune globulin and inactivated hepatitis B vaccination. Routine screening of all pregnant women and routine vaccination of all newborns is recommended.

HEPATITIS B IMMUNE GLOBULIN   AAP: Compatible
   Trade: H-Big, BayHep B, Nabi-HB
   Can/Aus/UK:
   Specifics: Immune globulin is 75% effective in preventing hepatitis B in sexual contacts when given prior to or within < 2 weeks after exposure to the virus.

HEPATITIS B VACCINATION   AAP: Compatible
   Trade: Recombivax HB, Energix-B
   Can/Aus/UK:
   Specifics: Inactivated hepatitis B vaccinations is >90%effective after three doses. A series of three doses given at 0, 1-2 months and 4-6 months is recommended. Vaccination is recommended IM in the deltoid muscle, not the buttocks.

INTERFERON Alfa-B   AAP: Not reviwed
Trade: Heberon Alfa R, Intron A
Can/Aus/UK:
Specifics: Interferon alfa-2b is an alpha interferon produced by recombinant DNA techniques. The typical duration of treatment is four to six months. Recommended dosing of Intron-A is 2.5 to 5 Million Units (MU) per meter square (/MSq) of body surface area three times a week. Higher doses (up to 10MU/MSq) of interferon may used with some benefit. The transfer of exogenously administered interferons into human milk is probably negligible as its molecular weight is quite large (> 20,000 daltons). Alfa N-3 interferon is known to pass poorly into human milk.
T1/2= 2-3 hours   Oral= N/A   Peak= 30 minutes

Clinical Tips:
Hepatitis B immune globulin is recommended for all infants born to mothers who are HbsAg-positive.   Routine vaccination of all newborns for hepatitis B is recommended.   In mothers positive for hepatitis B surface antigen, the infant can breastfeed if hepatitis immune globulin (HBIG 0.5 mL IM) and hepatitis B vaccination are given within 12 hours of birth. If the mothers Hepatitis B status is unknown, she should be tested immediately and the infant should receive the Hepatitis vaccine within 12 hours of birth.   If the mother tests positive, HBIG should be administered to the infant within 7 days of birth.   For the treatment of chronic Hepatitis B infections in breastfeeding patients, long-term interferon treatments may be required.   The transfer of these agents into milk is believed low due to their large molecular weight.   Interferon Alpha N3 has been studied in one patient and it levels in milk were unchanged following huge doses, suggesting these agents may not readily pass into milk.   More studies are desperately needed with the various interferons.

Suggested Reading:
1.   MMWR 1998 Guidelines for Teatment of Sexually Transmitted Disease.
2.   January 23, 1998 Vol/47No.RR-1 Recommendations and Reports.
3.   2002 Compenduium of Selected Publications The American College of OB/Gyn Women's Health Care Physicians, 2002.

Infectious Disease - Hepatitis C

Principles of Therapy:

Hepatitis C is a single-stranded RNA virus. Approximately 50% -70% of those with acute hepatitis C will develop chronic hepatitis C (HCV) and 20% of these will develop cirrhosis or chronic active disease. Risk factors for transmission are similar to those for hepatitis B, though sexual transmission appears to be significantly less effective than with hepatitis B. Only 15% of spouses without other risk factors have infection. Vertical transmission from mother to fetus occurs in 5 to 8 % of cases and is dependent on viral titer. Unlike hepatitis A or B, antibodies are not effective in preventing hepatitis C. No immune globulin or vaccination is presently available to prevent this infection. Anti-HCV and HCV-RNA have been detected in human milk. In a small study of 14 patients with HCV-RNA positive serum, only 2 had HCV-RNA positive breastmilk. Another small study of 15 HCV infected mothers who were HCV-RNA positive found that HCV-RNA was present in colostral samples though none of the 11 breastfed infants had HCV infection at 1 year of life. Breastfeeding in the scenario of maternal hepatitis C has not been documented to cause transmission to the infant in those patients which have been studied. In a study of 7,698 parturient women screened for anti-HCV antibodies, 53 were positive and of these 31 were HCV-RNA positive. Three of the 54 (5.6%) children born to these mothers became HCV-RNA positive during follow-up and all of these were from HCV-RNA positive mothers though breastfeeding was not evaluated. Another study from this same group in Japan found that in seven infected infants the mothers had significantly higher HCV-RNA titers.

Present data do not suggest a difference in transmission at 1 year of life between breastfed and formula fed infants suggesting that transmission of this infection via breastmilk is unlikely. The CDC and AAP consider maternal hepatitis C to be compatible with breastfeeding. In situations with a high maternal viral load use of artificial infant formula or banked milk if available may be a consideration. In another study of asymptomatic HCV positive mothers 2 of 87 infants (2.3%) became infected during follow-up. Two additional infected infants were born to women with chronic HCV infection. In all four of these cases the mother's HCV-RNA titers were > 5.0×10^6. Again, in these studies breastfeeding was not felt to be a risk factor but rather familial contact with the person with the high HCV-RNA titers. Treatment for chronic HCV infection with interferon therapy is associated with improvement in 28 to 46% of patients. Relapse rates, however, are as high as 50% within 6 months of completing therapy.

INTERFERON Alfa-2B + RIBAVIRIN   **AAP**: Not Reviewed
Trade: Rebetron
Can/Aus/UK:
Specifics: Rebetron is a combination of Interferon alfa-2B and ribavirin. While the transfer of interferons into milk is probably low to nil, there is some concern about the transfer of ribavirin into human milk.   Ribavirin concentrates in peripheral tissues and in the red blood cells in high concentrations over time (Vd= 802). Its elimination half-life at steady state averages 298 hours, which reflects slow elimination from nonplasma compartments. Red cell concentrations on average are 60 fold higher than plasma levels and may account for the occasional hemolytic anemia. It is likely the acute exposure of a breastfed infant would produce minimal side effects. However, chronic exposure over 12 months may be more risky, so caution is recommended.
T1/2= 298 hours   Oral= N/A   Peak= N/A
LRC = L4

Clinical Tips:
Maternal hepatitis C infection is compatable with breastfeeding with no documented increased risk of hepatitis C by one year of life for the infant.   The safety of breastfeeding in women with hepatitis C infection with a high viral load (HCV-RNA titer >5.0 x 10^6) is unclear. Adequate counseling with the patient in this particular situation is important. Measure of viral load may help to provide better-informed risk assessment. Maternal HCV-RNA titers > 5 x 10^6 may be associated with a higher mother-to-child transmission rate, but this may not be related to breastfeeding. Further investigation in this area is needed.   Some authorities recommend that that the mother who is HCV positive temporarily refrain from breastfeeding when there are cracked or bleeding nipples.

Suggested Reading:
1.   Moriya T. Transmission of hepatitis C virus from mothers to infants: its frequency and risk factors revisited. Biomed Pharmacother. 49(2): 59-64, January 1995.
2.   Gravovsky MO, et al. Hepatitis C Virus Infection in the Mothers and Infants Cohort Study. Pediatrics 102(2) August 1998.
3.   Manzini P. Human immunodeficiency virus infection as risk factor for mother-to-child hepatitis C virus transmission; persistence of anti-hepatitis C virus in children is associated with the mother's anti-hepatitis C virus immunoblotting pattern. Hepathology 21(2):328-32 February 1995.
4.   Lin HH. Absence of infection in breast-fed infants born to hepatitis C virus-infected mothers. Journal of Pediatrics 126(4) April 1995.
5.   Ohto H. Transmission of hepatitis C virus from mothers to infants. The Vertical Transmission of Hepatitis C Virus Collaborative Study Group. N Engl J Med 330 (1): 744-50. March 1994.
6.   Xiong H, Li B, Wu J. Detection of hepatitis C virus markers in colostrums. Zhonghua Fu Chan Ke ZA Zhi. 32 (3) 138-40, March 1997.

Infectious Disease - Herpes Simplex

Principles of Therapy:

Cutaneous herpes simplex virus infection is an incurable DNA viral infection that causes enlarging of infected epithelial cells, followed by nuclear degeneration and lysing of the cellular membrane. Some fuse to form the multinucleated giant cells typical of this infection. HSV-1 is most commonly found in the oropharynx while HSV-2 is most commonly associated with genital infections. Cross-over from this rule occurs, however, making specific HSV typing clinically rarely important. Diagnosis is best made using newer more sensitive methods such as PCR and hybridization techniques of suspected lesions. Samples should be taken from unroofed lesions. Serologic testing cannot reliably differentiate HSV 1 and HSV 2. Paired samples are required 2-3 weeks apart and are therefore not clinically helpful in guiding treatment. Genital HSV is usually acquired by sexual contact with a primary incubation period of 2 to 14 days and a duration of up to 21 days. Recurrent episodes typically last 5-7 days. Symptoms include fever, myalgia, inguinal adenopathy, bilateral vesicles followed by tender ulcers on the vulva and extensive cervicitis. The lesions are greyish in appearance, ulcerated and excruciatingly painful. Systemic symptoms are restricted to primary infections. Recurrent episodes are frequently preceded by prodromal symptoms which may be described as pain or tingling in the area prior to appearance of vulvar lesions. Treatment of recurrent episodes should be begun during prodrome or the first 24 hours after symptoms begin in order to be effective. Daily suppressive treatment can be given for patients with frequent outbreaks (6 or more outbreaks yearly). Antiviral medications do not eradicate the disease but are rather used for clinical benefit. Topical therapy for HSV is much less effective than oral therapy and its use is therefore discouraged.

ACYCLOVIR   **AAP**: Compatible
       Trade: Zovirax
       Can/Aus/UK: Zovirax, Avirax, Apo-Acyclovir, Acyclo-V, Zyclir, Aciclovir
       Specifics: Acyclovir is transferred into milk in low levels, approximating less than 1.5 mg per day. Percutaneous absorption from topical therapy is minimal.
       T1/2= 2.4 hours   Oral= 15-30%   Peak= 1.5 - 2 hours
       LRC= L2

FAMCYCLOVIR   **AAP**: Not Reviewed
       Trade: Famvir
       Can/Aus/UK: Famvir
       Specifics: Famciclovir is an antiviral use in the treatment of uncomplicated herpes zoster infection (shingles) and genital herpes. It is rapidly metabolized

to the active metabolite, penciclovir. Although similar to acyclovir, no data are available on levels in human milk. Oral bioavailability of famciclovir (77%) is much better than acyclovir (15-30%). Studies with rodents suggest that the milk/plasma ratio is greater than 1.0 but these seldom correlate with human data. Because famciclovir provides few advantages over acyclovir, at this point acyclovir would probably be preferred in a nursing mother although the side-effect profile is still minimal with this product.

T1/2= 2-3 hours   Oral= 77%   Peak= 0.9 hours
LRC= L2

VALACYCLOVIR   AAP: Not Reviewed
Trade: Valtrex
Can/Aus/UK:
Specifics: Valacyclovir is just a prodrug and is metabolized to acyclovir in the mother.
T1/2= 2.5-3 hours   Oral= 54%   Peak= 1.5 hours
LRC= L1

Clinical Tips:

The usefulness of acyclovir is largely determined by when it is used. If oral acyclovir is started early in the prodromal stage of infection, it may reduce the duration of shedding and time to healing by one-third. Treatment depends on if the infection is an initial symptomatic episode or a recurrence. First episodes are treated with either oral acyclovir 200mg five times daily or 400 mg three times daily, for 7 to 10 days. Alternatively, famciclovir 250mgs three times daily or valacyclovir 1 gm twice daily may be used for a similar duration. Recurrences are usually treated for 5 days. Acyclovir at similar doses as for first episode disease can be used or a dose of 800mgs twice daily can be given. Famciclovir 125mgs twice daily or valacyclovir 500mgs twice daily for five days are alternatives. Acyclovir is reasonably effective in suppressing recurrence if suppressive doses of 400 mg twice daily are maintained. Alternative suppressive therapies include famciclovir 250mgs twice daily or valacyclovir 500mgs or 1000mgs once daily. Suppressive therapy during breastfeeding may be less desirable than episodic treatment based on symptoms but would depend on the specific clinical situation. Valacyclovir is an ester of acyclovir which has improved oral absorption. Famcyclovir also has improved oral absorption. Perinatal infections with HSV are risky for the infant. While the primary mode of transmission to the infant is believed to be via the birth canal, transmission via contact with oropharyngeal and cutaneous lesions has been reported. Postnatally acquired infections can be equally lethal to those acquired during labor. A number of cases of herpes transmission via milk are reported. Caregivers should be urged to use strict cleanliness when providing care to the infant. Lesions directly on the breast should be covered prior to nursing. Lesions directly on the areola should preclude breastfeeding. Valcyclovir is frequently used due to its improved compliance with therapy as it does not require as frequent dosing.

Suggested Reading:

1. Whitley RJ, et al. Herpes simplex viruses. Clin Infect Dis. 1998 Mar;26(3):541-53;quiz 554-5. Review.
2. Schomogyi M, et al. Herpes simplex virus-2 infection. An emerging disease? Infect Dis Clin North Am. 1998 Mar;12(1):47-61. Review.
3. Klapper PE, et al. Herpes simplex virus. Intervirology. 1997;40(2-3):62-71. Review.
4. White C, et al. Genital herpes simplex infection in women. Clin Dermatol. 1997 Jan-Feb;15(1):81-91. Review.
5. MMWR 1998 Guidelines for Teatment of Sexually Transmitted Disease January 23, 1998 Vol/47No.RR-1 Recommendations and Reports.
6. 2002 Compenduium of Selected Publications The American College of OB/Gyn Women's Health Care Physicians, 2002.

Infectious Disease - Human Papilloma Virus

Principles of Therapy:

There are multiple different human papilloma virus types that cause warts. More than 20 different HPV types can cause infections of the genital tract. This can lead to either cervical dysplasia, genital warts or both, in addition to other less common problems. Though cervical cysplasia and condlyomata can be treated, the HPV can not be eradicated and vigilant long term follow-up is needed to detect recurrences. In compliant patients, mild cervical dysplasia can be followed as many cases will spontaneously regress. Treatment is indicated for suspected non-compliance, persistent, progressive or more advanced dysplasia. Cervical dysplasia treatment usually involves a destructive procedure such as cryotherapy or a loop electrosurgical excision procedure often referred to as a LEEP. These procedures would not commonly involve medications impacting the breastfeeding dyad. Cryotherapy can usually be performed in the office setting without medication. Occassionally, a paracervical block with lidocaine will be used for pain control for an office LEEP procedure. In other circumstances general anesthetic may be indicated for a day surgical procedure for a LEEP in an apprehensive or otherwise complicated patient. External vulvar warts can be treated by either provider applied therapy or by patient applied therapy. Choice of therapy depends largely on the size, location and number of lesions in addition to patient preference. With respect to effectiveness of therapy there is no single treatment that is superior. Provider applied therapies include: trichloroacetic acid (TCA), podophyllin, cryotherapy, interferon and surgical resection. Patient applied therapies include podofilox and imiquimod. Treatment requires repeated applications in most cases. Complications of therapy include pain and rarely scar formation.

IMIQUIMOD 5%   AAP: Not Reviewed
Trade: Aldara
Can/Aus/UK: Aldara
Specifics: Imiquimod is an immune response modifier useful for the treatment of external genital/perianal warts (venereal warts; condyloma acuminata). Imiquimod is typically applied three times weekly for up to 16 weeks. The area should be washed 6 to 10 hours after application. Imiquimod is virtually unabsorbed systemically. Plasma levels are undetectable. Transfer into milk is unlikely.
T1/2= N/A   Oral= N/A   Peak= N/A
LRC= L3

INTRALESIONAL INTERFERON Alfa-B   AAP: Not reviwed
Trade: Heberon Alfa R, Intron A
Can/Aus/UK:
Specifics: Interferon alfa-2b is an alpha interferon produced by recombinant

147

DNA techniques. The transfer of exogenously administered interferons particularly intralesional into human milk is probably negligible as its molecular weight is quite large (> 20,000 daltons). Alfa N-3 interferon is known to pass poorly into human milk.

T1/2= 2-3 hours   Oral= N/A   Peak= 30 minutes
LRC= L2

PODOFILOX 0.5%   AAP: Not Reviewed
Trade: Condylox
Can/Aus/UK: Condyline, Warticon
Specifics: Podofilox is an antimitotic agent used topically in the treatment of genital and perianal warts. Podofilox is applied to visible warts twice daily for three consecutive days followed by 4 days with no therapy. This may be repeated for 4 cycles.

T1/2= 1-4.5 hours   Oral= N/A   Peak= 1-2 hours
LRC= L3

PODOPHYLLIN RESIN 10% - 25%   AAP: Not Reviewed
Trade: Cascanyl, Pod-Ben-25, Podocon-25,
Can/Aus/UK: Canthacur-PS, Cantharone Plus
Specifics: Podophyllum resin is a naturally-occurring cytotoxic agent. A small amount is applied to warts with the patient instructed to wash the area 1 to 4 hours after treatment. This may be repeated weekly if needed. While systemic reactions have been reported with application to large areas, the use of this agent on limited areas is not contraindicated in breastfeeding infants.

T1/2= N/A   Oral=N/A   Peak= N/A
LRC = L3

TRICHLOROACETIC ACID 80% - 90%   AAP: Not Reviewed
Trade:
Can/Aus/UK:
Specifics: Trichloroacetic acid is a potent irritant and corrosive agent to the skin, eye and mucous membranes, but is not readily absorbed through the skin Trichloroacetic acid can denature protein and precipitate protein and may cause chemical burns to tissues which is basis for its use in treating warts. A small amount is applied directly to the wart until it becomes whitish. This may be repeated weekly if necessary.

T1/2= N/A   Oral= N/A   Peak= N/A

Clinical Tips:
Treatment for cervical dysplasia is unlikely to impact lactation. Various procedures are available which are locally destructive. Treatment of vulvar condylomata, however, may involve the use of topical medications. Condylomata may proliferate during pregnancy and regress spontaneously in the post-partum period. Treatment

may be given during pregnancy and cesarean delivery is rarely recommended unless the genital warts are obstructive. Persistent or newly occurring condylomata in the post-partum period would indicate treated. Cryotherapy would not impact the breastfed infant. Cryotherapy involves thermally induced cellular lyses and requires treatment in the physician's office with specialized equipment. Treatment may be painful and repeat therapy may be necessary. Surgical resection of condylomata can also be performed in the office setting under local anesthesia in some circumstances. Again, this would have minimal impact on lactation but can involve pain and scarring as possible consequences. Trichloroacetic acid is a locally caustic agent that induces a chemical cautery effect. Again, treatment requires an office visit and local extension of this liquid may cause damage to surrounding tissue. Minimal research has been done regarding the safety of podophyllin, podofilox and imiquimod during pregnancy and lactation. Podofilox and podophyllin are topical cytotoxic agent which cause arrest of mitosis. The podophyllin resin is frequently compounded with tincture of benzoin at strengths of 10-25%. Podophyllin requires careful application by the physician. Poisoning due to topical podophyllin application can occur. Most sources consider the use of podofilox and especially podophyllin to be contraindicated during pregnancy as safer alternatives are available though evidence of teratogenicity is limited. No data specific to lactation exists. Imiquimod in a topically active immune enhancing drug which stimulates local production of interferon and cytokines. Topical application results in minimal systemic absorption. Animal studies have not suggested imiquimod to be teratogenic and it is listed as category B for use during pregnancy.

Suggested Reading:

1. MMWR 1998 Guidelines for Teatment of Sexually Transmitted Disease January 23, 1998 Vol/47No.RR-1 Recommendations and Reports.
2. 2002 Compenduium of Selected Publications The American College of OB/Gyn Women's Health Care Physicians, 2002.

Infectious Disease
Intra-amniotic Infection / Post-partum
Endomyometritis

Principles of Therapy:

Intra-amniotic infection (also referred to as chorioamnionitis) is a relatively common infection during childbirth. It most likely occurs following prolonged rupture of membranes, long labors and multiple cervical examinations or intrauterine manipulation. Diagnostic criteria may include maternal fever, maternal leukocytosis, foul smelling or purulent amniotic fluid, maternal or fetal tachycardia and uterine tenderness. The infection occurs related to ascending organisms from vaginal flora in the vast majority of cases. Treatment for intra-amniotic infection includes the use of antibiotics and delivery of the infant. Infants born in the setting of this infection have increased morbidity and mortality. Antibiotics are typically continued intravenously for 24 (vaginal birth) to 48 (cesarean) hours after fever has resolved. Increased anaerobic bacterial coverage is typically added after a cesarean delivery. Post-partum endomyometritis (also referred to as metritis, endomyometritis, pelvic cellulites, endoparametritis, etc) is a similar infection that does not present until after delivery of the infant. The incidence of post-partum endomyometritis is increased in the patient who has undergone cesarean section. Prophylactic antibiotics are recommended at the time of cesarean section after the umbilical cord has been cut in an attempt to decrease infection risk. Infections tend to be polymicrobial and broad-spectrum antibiotics are generally recommended. As the infection is limited to the fetal membranes and the surrounding uterine tissues, breastfeeding and infant contact should not be of concern. The rare exception to this might be the critically ill mother with septicemia. In this situation, direct breastfeeding and contact with the infant would be impractical. Some typical antibiotic choices for the treatment of intra-amniotic infection and post-partum endomyometritis are listed below. The choice of other antibiotics may be appropriate in the particular setting. The vast majority of antibiotics are compatible with breastfeeding though the use of a fluoroquinolone would not be a first choice for this type of infection in a breastfeeding mother.

AMPICILLIN
AAP: Not Reviewed

Trade: Polycillin, Omnipen
Can/Aus/UK: Apo-Ampi, Novo-Ampicillin, NuAmpi, Penbriton, Ampicyn, Austrapen, Amfipen, Britcin, Vidopen
Specifics: Ampicillin levels in milk are generally less than 1 mg/Liter.
T½= 1.3 hours   Oral= 50%   Peak= 1-2 hours
LRC= L1

AMPICILLIN / SULBACTAM   AAP: Not Reviewed
Trade: Unasyn,
Can/Aus/UK: Magnapen
Specifics: Ampicillin+sulbactam is an antibiotic combination composed of ampicillin, and sulbactam, a beta-lactamase inhibitor. The addition of sulbactam extends the antimicrobial spectrum of ampicillin. Ampicillin levels in milk are generally less than 1 mg/Liter.
T½= 1.3 hours   Oral= 50%   Peak= 1-2 hours
LRC= L1

AZTREONAM   AAP: Compatible
Trade: Azactam
Can/Aus/UK: Azactam
Specifics: Following a single 1 g I.V. dose, breastmilk level was 0.18 mg/L at 2 hours and 0.22 mg/L at 4 hours. An infant would ingest approximately 33.0 µg/kg/day or < 0.03% of the maternal dose per day. The manufacturer reports that less than 1% of a maternal dose is transferred into milk. Due to poor oral absorption (<1%) no untoward effects would be expected in nursing infants, aside from changes in GI flora. Aztreonam is commonly used in pediatric units.
T½= 1.7 hours   Oral= <1%   Peak= 0.6-1.3 hours
LRC= L2

CEFOTETAN   AAP: Not Reviewed
Trade: Cefotan
Can/Aus/UK: Apatef, Cefotan
Specifics: Cefotetan is a third generation cephalosporin that is poorly absorbed orally and is only available via IM and I.V. injection. The drug is distributed into human milk in low concentrations. Following a maternal dose of 1000mg IM every 12 hours in 5 patients, breastmilk concentrations ranged from 0.29 to 0.59 mg/L. Plasma concentrations were almost 100 times higher. In a group of 2-3 women who received 1000 mg I.V., the maximum average milk level reported was 0.2 mg/L at 4 hours with a milk/plasma ratio of 0.02.
T1/2= 3-4.6 hours   Oral= Poor   Peak= 1.5 hours
LRC= L2

CEFOXITIN   AAP: Compatible
Trade: Mefoxin
Can/Aus/UK: Mefoxin
Specifics: Milk levels are very low, and oral bioavailability is poor. In a study of 2-3 women who received 1000 mg I.V., only trace amounts were reported in milk over 6 hours. In a group of 5 women who received an IM injection of 2000 mg, milk levels the highest milk levels were reported at 4 hours after dose. The maternal plasma levels varied from 22.5 at 2 hours to 77.6 µg/mL at 4 hours. Maternal milk levels ranged from < 0.25 to 0.65 mg/L.

151

T1/2= 0.7-1.1 hours   Oral= Poor   Peak= 20-30 min (IM)
LRC= L1

CLINDAMYCIN   AAP: Compatible
Trade: Cleocin
Can/Aus/UK: Dalacin, Clindatech, Cleocin
Specifics: Following oral doses of 300 mg every 6 hours, the breastmilk levels averaged 1.0 to 1.7 mg/L at 1.5 to 7 hours after dosing. One case of pseudomembranous colitis has been reported following high-dose IV therapy.
T1/2= 2.9 hours   Oral= 90%   Peak=45-60 min (oral)
LRC= L3

METRONIDAZOLE   AAP: May be of concern
Trade: Flagyl, Metizol, Trikacide, Protostat
Can/Aus/UK: Apo-Metronidazole, Flagyl, NeoMetric, Novo-Nidazol, Metrozine, Rozex
Specifics: Milk levels are low. Maximum reported levels are 15 µg/mL of milk. Infant's plasma levels are approximately 10% of maternal levels. No untoward effects have been reported in numerous studies.
T1/2= 8.5 hours   Oral= Complete   Peak= 2-4 hours
LRC= L2

GENTAMYCIN   AAP: Not Reviewed
Trade: Garamycin
Can/Aus/UK: Alocomicin, Cidomycin, Garamycin, Garatec,Palacos, Septopal
Specifics: The oral absorption of gentamicin (<1%) is generally nil with exception of premature neonates where small amounts may be absorbed. In one study of 10 women given 80 mg three times daily IM for 5 days postpartum, milk levels were measured on day 4. Gentamicin levels in milk were 0.42, 0.48, 0.49, and 0.41 mg/L at 1, 3, 5, and 7 hours respectively. The milk/plasma ratios were 0.11 at one hour and 0.44 at 7 hours. Plasma gentamicin levels in neonates were small, were found in only 5 of the 10 neonates, and averaged 0.41 µg/ml. The authors estimate that daily ingestion via breastmilk would be 307 µg for a 3.6 kg neonate (normal neonatal dose = 2.5 mg/kg every 12 hours).
T1/2= 2-3 hours   Oral= < 1%   Peak= N/A
LRC= L2

VANCOMYCIN   AAP: Not Reviewed
Trade: Vancocin
Can/Aus/UK: Vancocin, Vancoled
Specifics: Milk levels were 12.7 mg/L four hours after infusion in one woman receiving 1 gm every 12 hours for 7 days. Its poor absorption from the infant's GI tract would limit its systemic absorption.
T1/2= 5.6 hours   Oral= Minimal   Peak= N/A

LRC= L1

Clinical Tips:

Typical treatment of intra-amniotic infection often requires ampicillin (to cover Group B Strep) and gentamycin. Frequently clindamycin is added after cesarean delivery to provide improved anaerobic coverage. All three antibiotics are used for post-partum endomyometritis. These medications are often used in the immediate post-partum period by breastfeeding mothers without difficulty. The course of therapy is usually limited to a few days, typically 24 to 48 hours after the patient has defervesced. With the use of broad-spectrum antibiotics there is a theoretical risk of pseudomembranous colitis and observation for diarrhea is warranted. Vancomycin may be substituted for ampicillin in penicillin-allergic patients with endometritis.

Suggested Reading:

1.   2001 Compendium of Selected Publications The American College of OB/Gyn Women's Health Care Physicians, 2001.

Infectious Disease - Lyme Disease

Principles of Therapy:

Lyme disease is a systemic illness caused by the spirochete Borrelia burgdorferi. B. burgdorferi has been isolated from many tissues, including blood, skin, and cerebrospinal fluid. However, culture from the various sites is often inconclusive and a low-yield procedure. The primary mode of transmission is via tick bite. While common in the northeastern part of the USA, it also occurs commonly in Europe where it is transmitted by the sheep tick, Ixodes rincus. Within days to weeks following a tick bite, almost 80% of patients will have a red, expanding "bull's-eye" rash (called erythema migrans) accompanied by general fever, tiredness, headache, stiff neck, muscle aches and joint pain. If untreated, some patients may develop arthritis, including intermittent episodes of swelling and pain in the large joints; neurologic abnormalities such as aseptic meningitis, facial palsy, motor and sensory nerve inflammation (radiculoneuritis) and inflammation of the brain (encephalitis); and, rarely, cardiac problems such as atrioventricular block, acute inflammation of the tissues surrounding the heart (myopericarditis) or enlarged heart (cardiomegaly). The clinical features of lyme disease can be differentiated into three general stages: early localized, early disseminated, and later chronic infection. Acute infection with a vigorous inflammatory reaction is responsible for the most commonly observed clinical manifestations of Lyme disease. Features such as neurologic deficits and chronic arthritis occur much later and also respond poorly to treatment. It is not certain that live organisms are responsible for these late manifestations. Erythema migrans (erythematous macule or papule), the hallmark of Lyme disease, occurs at the site of tick bite generally within 3-32 days. While the lesion may be warm, pruritic and painful, it is often asymptomatic and easily missed. Spirochetes are readily cultured at this stage from the margins of the infection. Treatment largely depends on the stage of infection. Early infections respond effectively to penicillins, erythromycins, tetracyclines and cephalosporins.

AMOXICILLIN   AAP: Compatible

Trade: Larotid, Amoxil
Can/Aus/UK: Amoxil, Apo-Amoxi, Novamoxin, Alphamox, Moxacin, Cilamox, Betamox
Specifics: Amoxicillin levels in milk are low and average 0.9 mg/Liter of milk or lower.
T½= 1.7 hours   Oral= 89%   Peak= 1.5 hours
LRC= L1

AZITHROMYCIN   AAP: Not Reviewed

Trade: Zithromax
Can/Aus/UK: Zithromax
Specifics: Azithromycin levels in milk are very low.
T½= 48-68 hours   Oral= 37%   Peak= 3-4 hours
LRC=L2

CEFTRIAXONE   AAP: Not Reviewed
Trade: Rocephin
Can/Aus/UK: Rocephin
Specifics: Small amounts are transferred into milk (3-4% of maternal serum
level). Following a 1 gm IM dose, breastmilk levels were approximately 0.5-0.7
mg/L at between 4-8 hours. The estimated mean milk levels at steady state
were 3-4 mg/L. Another source indicates that following a 2 g/d dose and at
steady state, approximately 4.4 % of dose penetrates into milk. In this study,
the maximum breastmilk concentration was 7.89 mg/L after prolonged therapy
(7days). Using this data, the weight-adjusted relative infant dose would only be
0.35% of the maternal dose. Poor oral absorption of ceftriaxone would further
limit systemic absorption by the infant.
T½= 7.3 hours   Oral= Poor   Peak= 1 hour
LRC= L2

CEFUROXIME   AAP: Not Reviewed

Trade: Ceftin, Zinacef, Kefurox
Can/Aus/UK:
Specifics: Milk levels are believed to be low but are unreported.
T½= 1.4 hours   Oral= 30-50%   Peak= N/A
LRC= L2

DOXYCYCLINE   AAP: Not Reviewed

Trade: Doxychel, Vibramycin
Can/Aus/UK: Apo-Doxy, Doxycin, Vibramycin, Vibra-Tabs, Doryx,
Doxylin, Doxylar
Specifics: Milk levels are low (< 0.77 mg/L). Oral bioavailability is reduced
(20%) in milk but not eliminated. Limited use is unlikely to produce side
effects.
T½= 15-25 hours   Oral= 90-100%   Peak= 1.5-4 hours
LRC= L3
          L4 if used chronically

LYME DISEASE VACCINE   AAP: Not Reviewed

Trade: LYMErix
Can/Aus/UK:
Specifics: LYMErix is a noninfectious recombinant vaccine containing a lipoprotein from the outer surface of *Borrelia burgdorferi*. The lipoprotein from this causative agent is a single polypeptide chain of 257 amino acids with lipids covalently bonded to the N terminus. It is primarily indicated for individuals 15-70 years of age. It is very unlikely to enter milk. Officials from the CDC suggest that it is not contraindicated for use in breastfeeding patients.
LCR= L2

PENICILLIN G   AAP: Compatible

Trade: Pfizerpen
Can/Aus/UK:
Specifics: Milk levels vary from 7 to 60 units per liter following a dose of 100,000 units. Oral bioavailability is poor.
T½= <1.5 hours   Oral= 15-30%   Peak= 1-2 hours
LRC= L1

Clinical Tips:
According to the CDC, antibiotic treatment for 3-4 weeks with doxycycline or amoxicillin is generally effective in early disease. Treatment protocols for early lyme disease now consist of : Amoxicillin 500 mg t.i.d. X 21 days; Doxycycline 100 mg b.i.d. for 21 days; cefuroxime axetil 500 mg b.i.d. for 21 days; or azithromycin 500 mg daily for 7 days (less effective than prior regimens). Any of the above regimens are useful in breastfeeding women. Amoxicillin, cefuroxime, and azithromycin levels in breastmilk have been measured and are small. Loose stools or candida superinfections in the infant are possible. Doxycycline, while not ideal in breastfeeding mothers and their infants would not be a major problem when used for only 3 weeks. The absorption of doxycycline is reduced, though not eliminated, by calcium salts present in milk. For treatment of later manifestations such as arthritis or neurologic changes, similar antibiotics are used (ceftriaxone, penicillin G, doxycycline) except the doses are higher and more prolonged. Consult a current guide to antimicrobial therapy for further treatment protocols. Breastfeeding mothers can continue to nurse as soon as they are started on treatment.

The Lyme vaccine (LYMErix) is a noninfectious recombinant vaccine containing a lipoprotein from the outer surface of Borrelia burgdorferi. The lipoprotein from this causative agent is a single polypeptide chain of 257 amino acids with lipids covalently bonded to the N terminus. It is primarily indicated for individuals 15-70 years of age. It is very unlikely to enter milk. Officials from the CDC suggest that it is not contraindicated for use in breastfeeding patients.

Suggested Reading:

1. Evans J. Lyme disease. Curr Opin Rheumatol. 1998 Jul;10(4):339-46. Review.
2. Rahn DW, et al. Lyme disease update. Current approach to early, disseminated, and late disease. Postgrad Med. 1998 May;103(5):51-4, 57-9, passim. Review.
3. Keenan GF. Lyme disease: diagnosis & management. Compr Ther. 1998 Mar;24(3):147-52. Review.
4. Verdon ME, et al. Recognition and management of Lyme disease. Am Fam Physician. 1997 Aug;56(2):427-36, 439-40. Review.
5. CDC website: http://www.cdc.gov/ncidod/dvbid/lyme/

Infectious Disease - Malaria

Principles of Therapy:

Malaria is one of the oldest reported diseases. Symptoms include: history of exposure in a malaria-endemic area, periodic attacks of chills, fever and sweating, headache, myalgia, splenomegaly and anemia. Four Plasmodium species cause human malaria: Plasmodium vivax, P. malariae, P. ovale, and P. falciparum. Plasmodium vivax and falciparum account for most infections. The infective agent is the sporozoite, which is injected into the human by the bite of the mosquito. Treatment is separated into two modalities, prophylaxis treatment to prevent the disease or suppressive treatment to destroy the parasite. Treatment and prophylaxis have become increasingly difficult in recent years due to the spread of drug-resistant species. Resistance to chloroquine, primaquine and now mefloquine is growing rapidly and many regions of the world must depend on newer antimalarials for protection. Treating malaria appropriately requires knowledge of the infecting species, the location where the species was acquired and the geographic patterns of drug resistance. Treatment of malaria is two-fold, one is prophylaxis or prevention of infection, and two, to treat symptoms of prior or new infection. Fortunately, we have several good studies showing that the transfer of most antimalarials into human milk is quite low. Because infants who travel or live in these endemic areas must be prophylaxed anyway, the amount in breastmilk, which is small, is seldom relevant. For a complete review of medications used for malaria by country contact the Center for Disease Control.

ATOVAQUONE AND PROGUANIL   AAP: Not Reviewed

Trade: Malarone
Can/Aus/UK: Malarone
Specifics: Malarone is a fixed combination of atovaquone (250 mg) and proguanil (100 mg) (adult dose). Malarone is used both to prevent and treat malaria, particularly malaria resistant to certain other drugs. Both adult and pediatric formulations are available for treating pediatric patients down to 11 kg. There are no data available for transfer of these agents into human milk although the pharmaceutical company suggests that atovaquone concentrations in rodent milk were 30% of the concurrent concentrations in the maternal plasma. It is my experience that rodent levels are much higher than found in humans. Only trace quantities of proguanil were found in human milk. According to the CDC, breastfeeding mothers with infants less than 11 kg should use mefloquine instead of Malarone.
T½= N/A   Oral= N/A   Peak= N/A
LRC= L3 for infants > 11 kg

CHLOROQUINE   AAP: Compatible

Trade: Aralen, Novo-Chloroquine
Can/Aus/UK: Aralen, Chlorquin, Avloclor
Specifics: The amount of chloroquine in milk is very low. Following 5 mg/kg IM injection in lactating mothers 17 days postpartum, milk levels averaged 0.227 mg/L. In this study the milk level of chloroquine in 6 patients ranged from 0.192 to 0.319 mg/L. Based on these levels, the infant would consume approximately 34 µg/kg/day, an amount considered safe. Other studies have shown absorption to vary from 2.2 to 4.2% of maternal dose. The breastmilk concentration of chloroquine in this study averaged 0.58 mg/L following a single dose of 600 mg. Current recommended pediatric dose for patients exposed to malaria is 8.3 mg/kg per week.
T½= 72-120 hours   Oral= Complete   Peak= 1-2 hours
LRC= L3

DOXYCYCLINE   AAP: Not Reviewed

Trade: Doxychel, Vibramycin
Can/Aus/UK: Apo-Doxy, Doxycin, Vibramycin, Vibra-Tabs, Doryx, Doxylin, Doxylar
Specifics: Milk levels are low (< 0.77 mg/L). Oral bioavailability is reduced (20%) in milk but not eliminated. Limited use is unlikely to produce side effects. However, prolonged or repeated use over months is not recommended.
T½= 15-25 hours   Oral= 90-100%   Peak= 1.5-4 hours
LRC= L3
          L4 if used chronically

HYDROXYCHLOROQUINE   AAP: Compatible

Trade: Plaquenil
Can/Aus/UK: Plaquenil, Plaqueril
Specifics: Average milk concentration is 1.1 mg/Liter amounting to about 1/3 the clinical dose recommended for infants.
T½= >40 days   Oral= 74%   Peak= 1-2 hours
LRC= L2

MEFLOQUINE   AAP: Not Reviewed

Trade: Lariam
Can/Aus/UK: Lariam
Specifics: Milk concentrations are low, only 32-53 µg/liter of milk. Estimated ingestion by an infant would be approximately 0.14 mg/kg/day or about 3% of the maternal dose. According to the CDC, breastfeeding

mothers with infants less than 11 kg should use mefloquine instead of Malarone.

T½= 10-21 days.   Oral= 85%   Peak= 1-2 hours

LRC= L2

QUINIDINE   AAP: Compatible

Trade: Quinaglute, Quinidex

Can/Aus/UK: Apo-Quinidine, Cardioquin, Novo-Quinidin, Kinidin Durules, Kiditard

Specifics: Milk levels are quite low (<1% of dose). Because quinidine is stored in the liver, occasional liver enzyme studies in infant may be advisable after long-term exposure.

T½= 6-8 hours   Oral= 80%   Peak= 1-2 hours

LRC= L2

QUININE   AAP: Compatible

Trade: Quinamm

Can/Aus/UK:

Specifics: We have two good studies presently that show even after high doses, the amount of quinine in breastmilk is subclinical, less than 1-3 mg daily. Do not use concomitantly with digoxin.

T½= 11 hours   Oral= 76%   Peak= 1-3 hours

LRC= L2

PRIMAQUINE PHOSPHATE   AAP: Not Reviewed

Trade:

Can/Aus/UK:

Specifics: Milk levels have not been reported, but maternal plasma levels are incredibly low (< 107 ng/mL), suggesting milk levels would likely be low as well.

T½= 4-7 hours   Oral= 96%   Peak= 1-2 hours

LRC= L3

Clinical Tips:

Before any decision to treat or provide malaria prophylaxis is made, the clinician should closely review the excellent CDC website below for current recommendations.[6] Resistance of P. falciparum to chloroquine is widespread but in those areas where it is NOT resistant, once weekly doses of chloroquine are still effective. The clinical dose of chloroquine transferred via milk is quite low, only about 113 μg per day in mothers who received 5 mg/kg IM doses. This is minimal compared to the pediatric dose required for chemoprophylaxis (8.3 mg/kg/week). The amount of hydroxychloroquine transferred into milk is low as well, only about

1.1 mg per Liter of milk. The average infant would therefore ingest about 0.6 mg per day. Studies with mefloquine indicate that milk levels are very low, less than 53 µg per liter of milk. This is minimal compared to the prophylaxis dose of 4.6 mg/kg/week. Mefloquine is considered the drug of choice for chemoprophylaxis in children by the CDC. The CDC also recommends that mefloquine is preferred for breastfeeding mothers with infants less than 11 kg.

Doxycycline is a suitable choice for antimalarial prophylaxis in many parts of the world. While milk levels of doxycycline and oral bioavailability are low, long-term use (> 3 weeks) is probably not wise in breastfeeding mothers or children less than 8 years of age. Quinine transfer into milk is extremely low and is unlikely to be clinically relevant. Estimated transfer of quinine varies with dose but would likely be less than 1-3 mg daily. In places where quinine is not available, quinidine may be substituted. Quinidine transfer into milk is believed less than 6.4 mg/liter of milk. This would be significantly less than pediatric therapeutic doses.

Suggested Reading:

1.   Makler MT, et al. A review of practical techniques for the diagnosis of malaria. Ann Trop Med Parasitol. 1998 Jun;92(4):419-33. Review.
2.   Clark IA, et al. The biological basis of malarial disease. Int J Parasitol. 1997 Oct;27(10):1237-49. Review.
3.   Krishna S. Science, medicine, and the future. Malaria. BMJ. 1997 Sep 20;315(7110):730-2. Review.
4.   Stanley J. Malaria. Emerg Med Clin North Am. 1997 Feb;15(1):113-55. Review.
5.   Murphy GS, et al. Falciparum malaria. Infect Dis Clin North Am. 1996 Dec;10(4):747-75. Review.
6.   CDC website: http://www.cdc.gov/ncidod/dpd/parasites/malaria/default.htm

Infectious Disease - Salmonellosis

Principles of Therapy:

Salmonellosis includes infection by any of 2000 serotypes of salmonellae. Human infections are generally caused by one of three major subtypes, S. typhi, typhimurium, and choleraesuis. Three clinical patterns of infections are most common and include: enteric fever (typhoid fever caused by S. typhi); acute enterocolitis (S. typhimurium); and bacterial septicemia (S. choleraesuis). All such infections are due to the ingestion of contaminated food or drink. Treatment depends on the subtype of infection.

AMPICILLIN   AAP: Not Reviewed

Trade: Polycillin, Omnipen
Can/Aus/UK: Apo-Ampi, Novo-Ampicillin, NuAmpi, Penbriton, Ampicyn, Austrapen, Amfipen, Britcin, Vidopen
Specifics: Ampicillin levels in milk are generally less than 1 mg/Liter.
T½= 1.3 hours   Oral= 50%   Peak= 1-2 hours
LRC= L1

CEFIXIME   AAP: Not Reviewed

Trade: Suprax
Can/Aus/UK:
Specifics: Milk levels are low, often undetectable. It is secreted to a limited degree in the milk, although in one study of a mother receiving 100 mg, it was undetected in the milk from 1-6 hours after the dose.
T½= 7 hours   Oral= 30-50%   Peak= 2-6 hours
LRC= L2

CEFOPERAZONE SODIUM   AAP: Not Reviewed

Trade: Cefobid
Can/Aus/UK:
Specifics: Following high IV doses, milk levels were less than 0.9 mg/Liter of milk.
T½= 2 hours   Oral= Poor   Peak= 73-153 min.(IV)
LRC= L2

CEFOTAXIME   AAP: Compatible

Trade: Claforan
Can/Aus/UK: Claforan
Specifics: Milk levels are very small, less than 0.32 mg/Liter of milk.
T½= < 0.68 hr.   Oral= Poor   Peak= 30 min.
LRC= L2

CEFTRIAXONE   AAP: Not Reviewed
Trade: Rocephin
Can/Aus/UK: Rocephin
Specifics: Small amounts are transferred into milk (3-4% of maternal serum level). Following a 1 gm IM dose, breastmilk levels were approximately 0.5-0.7 mg/L at between 4-8 hours. The estimated mean milk levels at steady state were 3-4 mg/L. Another source indicates that following a 2 g/d dose and at steady state, approximately 4.4 % of dose penetrates into milk. In this study, the maximum breastmilk concentration was 7.89 mg/L after prolonged therapy (7days). Using this data, the weight-adjusted relative infant dose would only be 0.35% of the maternal dose. Poor oral absorption of ceftriaxone would further limit systemic absorption by the infant.
T½= 7.3 hours   Oral= Poor   Peak= 1 hour
LRC= L2

CIPROFLOXACIN   AAP: Approved

Trade: Cipro, Ciloxan
Can/Aus/UK: Cipro, Ciloxan, Ciproxin
Specifics: In one study of 10 women who received 750 mg every 12 hours, milk levels of ciprofloxacin ranged from 3.79 mg/L at 2 hours post-dose to 0.02 mg/L at 24 hours. In another study of a single patient receiving one 500 mg tablet daily at bedtime, the concentrations in maternal serum and breastmilk were 0.21 µg/mL, and 0.98 µg/mL, respectively. Plasma levels were undetectable (< 0. 03 µg/mL) in the infant. The dose to the 4 month old infant was estimated to be 0.92 mg/day or 0.15 mg/kg/day. No adverse effects were noted in this infant. There has been one reported case of severe pseudomembranous colitis in an infant of a mother who self-medicated with ciprofloxacin for 6 days.
T½= 4.1 hours   Oral= 50-85%   Peak= 0.5-2.3 hours
LRC= L4

FURAZOLIDONE   AAP: Not Reviewed

Trade: Furoxone
Can/Aus/UK:
Specifics: Poor oral bioavailability. Milk levels are unreported.
T½= N/A   Oral= < 5%   Peak= N/A
LRC= L3

OFLOXACIN   AAP: Not Reviewed

Trade: Floxin
Can/Aus/UK: Floxin, Ocuflox, Tarivid
Specifics: In one study in lactating women who received 400 mg oral doses twice daily, drug concentrations in breastmilk averaged 0.05-2.41 mg/L in milk (24 hours and 2 hours post-dose respectively). Milk levels are much lower than ciprofloxacin levels.
T½= 5-7 hours   Oral= 98 %   Peak= 0.5-2 hours
LRC= L3

CO-TRIMOXAZOLE   AAP: Compatible

Trade: TMP-SMZ, Bactrim, Cotrim, Septra
Can/Aus/UK: Novo-Trimel, Septrin, Bactrim, Respax, Trimogal
Specifics: Mixture of trimethoprim and sulfamethoxazole. Trimethoprim levels vary from 1.2-5.5 mg/liter of milk.
T½= N/A   Oral= N/A   Peak= N/A
LRC= L3

TROVAFLOXACIN MESYLATE   AAP: Not Reviewed

Trade: Trovan, Alatrofloxacin
Can/Aus/UK:
Specifics: Reported milk levels are very low and averaged 0.8 mg/Liter of milk. Recent data suggest this product may be hepatotoxic and caution is recommended.
T½= 12.2 hours   Oral= 88%   Peak= 1-2 hours
LRC= L4

Clinical Tips:

Enteric fever (Typhoid Fever) may be caused by any of the Salmonella species. Currently, due to the emergence of high resistance, ampicillin and chloramphenicol are seldom recommended. Trimethoprim-sulfamethoxazole (TMP/SMX) is generally preferred. Of the cephalosporins, ceftriaxone (2 gm daily) for 3-7 days is quite effective. Other effective cephalosporins include cefixime, cefotaxime and cefoperazone. The fluoroquinolones, although not ideal in breastfeeding mothers, can be used with caution particularly ofloxacin. Duration of therapy is 5-7 days. Due to lower milk levels, ofloxacin and trovafloxacin are preferred. Acute enterocolitis is the most common salmonella infection. Fluid and electrolyte therapy remains the best initial treatment as most cases are self-limited. Antimotility drugs such as loperamide or diphenoxylate should be discouraged as they may increase complications and lead to bacteremia. Antibiotics are generally not needed for the uncomplicated salmonella enterocolitis in normal patients. However, in patients with co-morbid conditions such as immunodeficiency states(HIV), then TMP/SMX or the fluoroquinolones as above are preferred. Treatment of salmonellosis with antibiotics, if possible, should be avoided as it frequently leads to a permanent carrier state.

Suggested Reading:

1. Gomez TM, et al. Foodborne salmonellosis. World Health Stat Q. 1997;50(1-2):81-9. Review.
2. Tietjen M, et al. Salmonellae and food safety. Crit Rev Microbiol. 1995;21(1):53-83. Review.

Infectious Disease - Syphilis

Principles of Therapy:

Syphilis is caused by the spirochete Treponema pallidum. The presentation of this disease varies over time. Primary syphilis manifests as a painless ulcer (chancre) usually 1 month after exposure that then spontaneously heals in 1 to 2 months. This often goes undiagnosed in women. Presentation of secondary syphilis may involve a rash typically noted on the palm and soles, condylomata lata (velvet like vulvar lesions), lymphadenopathy, fever and malaise. This occurs from one to six months after the initial chancre. Spontaneous regression occurs after one month but tertiary syphilis may then present many years later if left untreated. Effects related to tertiary syphilis include skin lesions, aortic aneurysm, tabes dorsales (CNS lesions) and bone lesions (gummas). Diagnosis of primary syphilis can be done using dark field microscopy or direct fluorescent antibody tests of exudates from the lesion. Blood testing is ineffective for primary syphilis. Serologic testing can be done with either a VDRL or RPR test. A confirmatory MHA-TP test is indicated to confirm diagnosis as the other tests are indirect and can be falsely positive. VDRL or RPR titers are used in monitoring therapy over time. Treatment involves the use of Benzathine penicillin G.

BENZATHINE PENICILLIN G   AAP: Not Reviewed
    Trade: Bicillin
    Can/Aus/UK:
    Specifics: Benzathine penicillin is the prolonged release formulation of penicillin G. While no data are available on the transfer of this form of penicillin, following IM doses of 100,000 units of procain penicillin G, the milk/plasma ratios varied between 0.03-0.13. Milk levels varied from 7 units to 60 units/L.
    T1/2= hours   Oral= Poor   Peak= N/A
    LRC= L1

Clinical Tips:

The only proven effective treatment for syphilis is penicillin G. During pregnancy no alternative is acceptable and penicillin allergic patients should be desensitized to allow for penicillin therapy. Non-pregnant penicillin allergic patients can be treated with oxycycline 100mgs twice daily, or tetracycline 500mgs four times daily for two weeks. Treatment with penicillin G is preferred and this would be of little concern for lactation. Primary and secondary syphilis can be treated with a single injection of 2.4 million units of penicillin G intramuscularly. This single injection is also used for treatment of early latent disease. Early latent disease is diagnosed when there is no demonstrable evidence of disease but the serologic testing is now positive and was known to be negative within the preceding year. Late latent disease or disease present for an unknown duration is treated with three weekly injections of

2.4 million units of penicillin G for a total of 7.2 million units. Most breastfeeding women and newborn infants would have had serologic testing done at the time of delivery in the United States. It is likely that the breastfed infant will require treatment for syphilis as well and the infant should be referred for evaluation

Suggested Reading:
1.   MMWR 1998 Guidelines for Teatment of Sexually Transmitted Disease January 23, 1998 Vol/47No.RR-1 Recommendations and Reports.

Infectious Disease – Trichomoniasis

Principles of Therapy:

Trichomoniasis is a vaginal infection caused by the flagellated protozoan, Trichomonas vaginalis. While most common in women, it can infect the bladder and urethra of men as well and can be sexually transmitted. Trichomoniasis is frequently asymptomatic in both women and men although 50-75% of infected women complain of a frothy off-white, purulent green or yellow vaginal discharge. There may be a fishy amine odor as well as itching, irritation, dyspareunia and dysuria. The diagnosis is established by visualizing the mobile protozoan in a saline preparation of vaginal secretions under the microscope. Effective therapy is limited to oral metronidazole. Metronidazole gel is useful for treatment of bacterial vaginosis but is less effective than oral metronidazole for trichomonas and is not recommended. Although somewhat less effective, intravaginal clotrimazole suppositories or povidone vaginal douches may be effective, but are not preferred in pregnant or breastfeeding women. Male sexual partners should be treated as well. Resistance to metronidazole is rising and may require special treatment regimens.

CLOTRIMAZOLE   AAP: Not Reviewed
Trade: Gyne-Lotrimin, Mycelex, Lotrimin, Femcare
Can/Aus/UK: Canesten, Clotrimaderm, Myclo, Clonea, Hiderm
Specifics: Systemic absorption following intravaginal use in minimal (< 3-10%).
T1/2= 3.5-5 hours   Oral= Poor   Peak= 3 hours (oral)
LRC= L1

METRONIDAZOLE   AAP: May be of concern
Trade: Flagyl, Metizol, Trikacide, Protostat
Can/Aus/UK: Apo-Metronidazole, Flagyl, NeoMetric, Novo-Nidazol, Metrozine, Rozex
Specifics: Milk levels are low. Maximum reported levels are 15 µg/mL of milk. Infant's plasma levels are approximately 10% of maternal levels. No untoward effects have been reported in numerous studies.
T1/2= 8.5 hours   Oral= Complete   Peak= 2-4 hours
LRC= L2

Clinical Tips:

Effective treatment is generally limited to oral therapy with metronidazole. Two regimens are generally used, a one-time 2 gram STAT dose of metronidazole or 500 mg twice daily for 7 days. The 2-gram dose is about 95% effective in women. Because the effectiveness of the single dose regimen in males is unclear, male partners should be treated with the 500 mg dose twice daily for 7 days unless non-compliance is a concern. Retreatment using metronidazole 500 mgs twice daily is recommended for initial failures. Although human data has found that metronidazole is not dangerous to a fetus, there is a relative contraindication to using metronidazole in the first trimester of pregnancy. Use in breastfeeding mothers is similarly controversial although this is largely unfounded. Metronidazole transfer into human milk is moderate to low. Several treatment regimens can be recommended. The 2-gram STAT dose, followed by pumping and discarding of milk for 12-24 hours is preferred. At 12 hours, the maternal plasma levels of metronidazole are approaching the trough. At 24 hours, the reported peak dose of metronidazole via milk (following a 2000 mg maternal dose) would be less than 10 mg per liter of milk. Thus far, no reports of untoward effects have been found following the use of this protocol in breastfeeding mothers. Alternate protocols, such as 400 mg three times daily have also been studied. The dose to the infant via milk was less than 15 mg per liter of milk. While most infants ingest far less than a liter of milk daily (estimated intake =150ml/kg), the dose received by the infant would be correspondingly lower. Other recommended doses include 250 mg three times daily or 500 mg twice daily. Metronidazole may induce disulfiram-like reactions with alcohol, unusual metallic taste and darkened urine. While metronidazole is not FDA approved for pediatric use, the published pediatric dose in term infants is 15 mg/kg/day. In those patients unable to take metronidazole, clotrimazole vaginal suppositories may be effective. Other therapies, although less effective, include an antitrichomonal suppository (e.g. Vagisec Plus [polyoxyethylene nonyl phenol, aminacrine, sodium edetate, and docusate sodium]). While povidone iodine douches have been use in the past, they may lead to significant absorption of iodine by the mother and breastfeeding infant. If used, they should only be used briefly.

Suggested Reading:

1. Gulmezoglu AM, et al. Trichomoniasis treatment in women: a systematic review. Trop Med Int Health. 1998 Jul;3(7):553-8. Review.
2. Ries AJ. Treatment of vaginal infections: candidiasis, bacterial vaginosis, and trichomoniasis. J Am Pharm Assoc (Wash). 1997 Sep-Oct;NS37(5):563-9. Review.
3. MMWR 1998 Guidelines for Teatment of Sexually Transmitted Disease January 23, 1998 Vol/47No.RR-1 Recommendations and Reports.

Infectious Disease – Tuberculosis

Principles of Therapy:

The incidence of tuberculosis is rising, due to the emergence of HIV/AIDS, immigration of people from areas with a high prevalence of tuberculosis, increased poverty and homelessness among this population, and a deterioration of health care systems which previously monitored tuberculosis care. Diagnosis is more or less straightforward with the Mantoux tuberculin skin test, chest radiographs and sputum cultures. Symptoms include: fatigue, weight loss, fever, night sweats, productive cough and pulmonary infiltrates on chest radiograph. The Mantoux skin test (PPD) is highly predictive of infection with mycobacterium tuberculosis (MTB), as judged by the size of the induration surrounding the injection site. The treatment of MTB has become increasingly difficult with the emergence of multidrug resistant strains. Multidrug therapy is the standard, using isoniazid, rifampin, pyrazinamide initially, followed in 2 months by isoniazid and rifampin (one of many regimens). Ethambutol or streptomycin is reserved for resistant species. Most of the anti-tubercular drugs pass into milk, but the levels transmitted are generally less than 20% of the therapeutic (pediatric) dose used in children, and thus far has not been reported to be a major problem in breastfed infants. Mothers can continue to breastfeed according to the American Academy of Pediatrics while undergoing isoniazid or rifampin therapy.

CYCLOSERINE   **AAP**: Compatible

> **Trade:**   Seromycin
> **Can/Aus/UK:**
> **Specifics:**   Levels in milk range from 6 to 19 mg per liter.
> T½= 12+ hours   Oral= 70-90%   Peak= 3-4 hours
> LRC= L3

ETHAMBUTOL   **AAP**: Compatible

> **Trade:**   Ethambutol, Myambutol
> **Can/Aus/UK:** Etibi, Myambutol
> **Specifics:**   Ethambutol levels in milk are reported low, less than 4.6 mg per liter of milk.
> T½= 3.1 hours   Oral= 80%   Peak= 2-4 hours
> LRC= L2

ISONIAZID   AAP: Compatible

Trade: INH, Laniazid
Can/Aus/UK:
Specifics: Isoniazid levels in milk are controversial, and range from 6 to 16.6 mg per liter of milk. The pediatric half-life is longer than adults and some elevated neonatal plasma levels have been reported. Attempt to breastfeed at times when maternal peak levels are lowest.
T½= 1.1 – 3.1 hours   Oral= Complete   Peak= 1-2 hours(oral)
LRC= L3

RIFAMPIN   AAP: Compatible

Trade: Rifadin, Rimactane
Can/Aus/UK: Rifadin, Rimactane, Rofact, Rifampicin, Rimycin
Specifics: Reported milk levels are very low, only 3.4 to 4.9 mg per liter of milk.
T½= 3.5 hours   Oral= 90-95%   Peak= 2-4 hours
LRC= L2

STREPTOMYCIN   AAP: Compatible

Trade:
Can/Aus/UK:
Specifics: Streptomycin levels in milk are very low, less than 0.6 mg per liter of milk. The oral bioavailability of streptomycin is extremely poor.
T½= 2.6 hours   Oral= Poor   Peak= 1-2 hours (IM)
LRC= L3

PYRAZINAMIDE   AAP: Not Reviewed

Trade: Pyrazinamide
Can/Aus/UK:
Specifics: Peak milk levels are 1.5 mg per liter of milk following a 1 gm dose.
T½= 9-10 hours   Oral= Complete   Peak= 2 hours
LRC= L3

Clinical Tips:

Initial therapy for individuals with positive PPD screens is chemoprophylaxis with Isoniazid (INH) 300mg/day for 6 to 9 months for adults. Chemoprophylaxis is primarily for individuals whose PPD skin test has converted from negative to positive within the last 2 years. Isoniazid passes into human milk in low levels, but over an extended time, may produce moderate plasma levels in some infants. Infants should periodically be monitored for elevated INH plasma levels and liver transaminases. Breastfeeding should be scheduled to avoid the peak maternal plasma levels at 1-3 hours post dose. This will significantly reduce exposure of the infant to higher breastmilk levels. Maternal pyridoxine therapy (B-6 10 mg daily) is recommended. Rifampin levels in breastmilk have been reported and are quite low. Following a 450 mg dose, milk levels were less than 4.9 mg per liter. Following a 600 mg dose, peak milk levels were 10-30 mg per liter. Streptomycin is a first line choice for treatment of rapidly multiplying bacilli. While it can induce significant VIII cranial nerve damage and deafness, its breastmilk levels are very low. Further, its oral bioavailability is virtually nil. Cycloserine works similarly to ethambutol. Its milk levels range to a peak as high as 19 mg per liter following a 250 mg maternal dose. Pyrazinamide is commonly used as an Option 1 drug, and is used in combination with isoniazid and rifampin. Reported milk levels of pyrazinamide (peak) are low at only 1.5 mg per liter of milk. Current CDC recommendations for treating TB are: Option 1 = Isoniazid, Rifampin, and pyrazinamide; Option 2 = Isoniazid, Rifampin, Pyrazinamide, and Streptomycin or Ethambutol. Please refer to the CDC guidelines for complete recommendations, including treatment of multi-drug resistant forms.

Suggested Reading:

1. Woeltje KF. Tuberculosis: what you don't know can hurt you. Infect Control Hosp Epidemiol. 1998 Sep;19(9):626-8. Review.
2. Albino JA, et al. The treatment of tuberculosis. Respiration. 1998;65(4):237-55. Review.
3. Zumla A, et al. Tuberculosis. BMJ. 1998 Jun 27;316(7149):1962-4. Review.
4. Brandli O.The clinical presentation of tuberculosis. Respiration. 1998;65(2):97-105. Review.
5. CDC website: http://www.cdc.gov/nchstp/tb/faqs/qa.htm#Introduction

Infectious Disease – Varicella

Principles of Therapy:

Varicella (chickenpox or shingles) is caused by the varicella-zoster DNA herpes virus. It is very contagious and is spread by contact with vesicular fluid or respiratory droplets. This is a common disease of childhood during which time the vast majority of infections are minor self-limited infections. During adulthood and especially pregnancy the risk of more serious complications from this infection increases. Immunosuppression also increases the risk associated with this infection. Incubation varies from 10 to 21 days after exposure until lesions appear. If a known exposure has occurred it is possible to give post-exposure vaccination to a breastfeeding woman. Routine vaccination of children between 12 and 18 months of life is now given. Women of childbearing potential who have no history of chickenpox should be offered testing and vaccination prior to pregnancy. As the vaccination is a live attenuated virus it should not be given within one month preceding or during pregnancy. A critical time period for this infection to occur is within 5 days prior to or 48 hours after delivery of the infant. This allows potential transmission of the virus but not maternal antibodies to the infant. Infants born to mothers with active varicella should be isolated from mother and given varicella zoster immune globulin (VZIG).

VARICELLA ZOSTER IMMUNE GLOBULIN   AAP: Compatible
Trade: Varicella Zoster Immune Globulin
Can/Aus/UK:
Specifics: Varicella-Zoster immune globulin (Human) (VZIG) is a human globulin fraction (primarily IgG). As a large molecular weight protein, it would not likely transfer into human milk past the first 48 hours postpartum. It is commonly used in infants.
T1/2= 3 weeks.   Oral= Poor   Peak= N/A
LRC= L1

VARICELLA ZOSTER VACCINATION   AAP: Not Reviewed
Trade: Varivax
Can/Aus/UK:
Specifics: Varicell Zoster vaccine is a live attenuated vaccine indicated for the prevention of varicella. It is cleared for use in children > 12 months of age although it is commonly used in infants. Both the AAP and the Center for Disease Control approve the use of varicella-zoster vaccines in breastfeeding mothers, if the risk of infection is high.
T1/2= 1.2-2.2 hours   Oral= Poor   Peak= 1-2 hours
LRC= L2

Clinical Tips:

Infants born to mothers with active chickenpox at delivery should be isolated from other infants and given VZIG. It is unclear if transmission via breastmilk can occur but spread by contact is well documented. Ideally, in breastfeeding mothers exposed to infection, post-exposure vaccination can be given potentially avoiding both maternal chickenpox and any disruption in lactation. For breastfed infants greater than one year of age vaccination of the child itself is recommended. Shingles should not provide a concern for breastfeeding provided that the lesions can be adequately covered to avoid contact with the infant. VZIG may also be given to the infant in cases of maternal shingles as a precaution.

Suggested Reading::

1.   Frederick IB, White RJ, et.al. Excretion of varicella-herpes zoster virus in breast milk. Am. J. Obstet. Gynecol. 154:1116-7, 1986.
2.   American Academy of Pediatrics. Committee on Infectious Diseases. Red Book 1997.

Infectious Disease – Wound Infection

Principles of Therapy:

Wound infections frequently occur with an incidence of approximately 4 to 12 % of patients undergoing cesarean delivery. Typically wound infections present 4 to 5 days after surgery. The wound is found to be erythematous and tender. Fever may also be present. Treatment involves opening, draining, debriding and cleaning of the wound. Various techniques are used to assist with wound healing. Some advocate the use of secondary closure of the wound after the infection has been cleared, while others recommend healing by secondary intent and the use of vacuum devices. Antibiotics typically used to treat wound infections should have coverage for staphylococcus and streptococcus species. Again, many different antibiotics may be used for this common infection. Oral or intravenous antibiotics may be chosen depending on the clinical situation. Some of the commonly used antibiotics for wound infections are listed below.

AMOXICILLIN + CLAVULANATE   **AAP:** Compatible

Trade: Larotid, Amoxil
Can/Aus/UK: Amoxil, Apo-Amoxi, Novamoxin, Alphamox, Moxacin, Cilamox, Betamox
Specifics: Amoxicillin levels in milk are low and average 0.9 mg/Liter of milk or lower. Current studies show amoxicillin by itself is no more effective than placebo in infectious sinusitis.
T½= 1.7 hours   Oral= 89%   Peak= 1.5 hours
LRC= L1

CEFAZOLIN   **AAP:** Approved
Trade: Ancef, Kefzol
Can/Aus/UK: Ancef, Kefzol, Cefamezin
Specifics: In 20 patients who received a 2 gm STAT dose over 10 minutes, the average concentration of cefazolin in milk in 2, 3, and 4 hours after the dose was 1.25, 1.51, and 1.16 mg/L, respectively.
T1/2= 1.2-2.2 hours   Oral= Poor   Peak= 1-2 hours
LRC= L1

CEFOTETAN   **AAP:** Not Reviewed
Trade: Cefotan
Can/Aus/UK: Apatef, Cefotan
Specifics: Cefotetan is a third generation cephalosporin that is poorly absorbed orally and is only available via IM and I.V. injection. The drug is distributed into human milk in low concentrations. Following a maternal dose of 1000mg IM every 12

hours in 5 patients, breastmilk concentrations ranged from 0.29 to 0.59 mg/L. Plasma concentrations were almost 100 times higher. In a group of 2-3 women who received 1000 mg I.V., the maximum average milk level reported was 0.2 mg/L at 4 hours.
T1/2= 3-4.6 hours Oral= Poor   Peak= 1.5 hours
LRC= L1

CEFOXITIN   AAP: Compatible
Trade: Mefoxin
Can/Aus/UK: Mefoxin
Specifics: Milk levels are very low, and oral bioavailability is poor. In a study of 2-3 women who received 1000 mg I.V., only trace amounts were reported in milk over 6 hours. In a group of 5 women who received an IM injection of 2000 mg, the highest milk levels were reported at 4 hours after dose. The maternal plasma levels varied from 22.5 at 2 hours to 77.6 µg/mL at 4 hours. Maternal milk levels ranged from < 0.25 to 0.65 mg/L.
T1/2= 0.7-1.1 hours Oral= Poor Peak= 20-30 min (IM)
LRC= L1

CEPHALEXIN   AAP: Approved
Trade: Keflex
Can/Aus/UK: Apo-Cephalex, Ceporex, Novo-Lexin, Ibilex, Keflex
Specifics: Following a 1000 mg maternal oral dose, milk levels at 1, 2, 3, 4, and 5 hours ranged from 0.20, 0.28, 0.39, 0.50, and 0.47 mg/L respectively. Milk/serum ratios varied from 0.008 at 1 hour, to 0.140 at 3 hours. These levels are probably too low to be clinically relevant.
T1/2= 50-80 minutes Oral= Complete Peak= 1 hour
LRC= L1

DICLOXACILLIN   AAP:
Trade: Pathocil, Dycill, Dynapen
Can/Aus/UK: Diclocil
Specifics: Following oral administration of a 250 mg dose, milk concentrations of the drug were 0.1, and 0.3 mg/L at 2 and 4 hours after the dose, respectively. Levels were undetectable after 6 hours.
T1/2= 0.6-0.8 hours Oral= 35-76% Peak= 0.5-2 hours
LRC= L1

CLINDAMYCIN   AAP: Approved
Trade: Cleocin
Can/Aus/UK: Dalacin, Clindatech, Cleocin
Specifics: Following oral doses of 300 mg every 6 hours, the breastmilk levels averaged 1.0 to 1.7 mg/L at 1.5 to 7 hours after dosing. One case of pseudomembranous colitis has been reported following high-dose IV therapy.
T1/2= 2.9 hours Oral= 90% Peak=45-60 min (oral)

LRC= L3

NAFCILLIN
Trade: Unipen, Nafcil
Can/Aus/UK: Unipen
Specifics: No data are available on the concentration of nafcillin in milk but it is likely small. Oral absorption in the infant would be minimal.
T1/2= 0.5-1.5 hours   Oral= 50%   Peak= 30-60 min(IM)
LRC= L1

VANCOMYCIN
Trade: Vancocin
Can/Aus/UK: Vancocin, Vancoled
Specifics: Milk levels were 12.7 mg/L four hours after infusion in one woman receiving 1 gm every 12 hours for 7 days. Its poor absorption from the infant's GI tract would limit its systemic absorption.
T1/2= 5.6 hours   Oral= Minimal   Peak= N/A
LRC= L1

Clinical Tips:
Antibiotics are not required in all cases of wound infections. The clinical situation dictates when wound care is sufficient, but in some situations oral or intravenous antibiotics may be needed to treat cellulitis. Many antibiotics provide adequate coverage for the suspected organisms and are compatible with breastfeeding. Avoidance of the fluoroquinolone type of antibiotics is preferable.

Suggested Reading:
1. Yamaguchi Y, Yoshikawa K. Cutaneous wound healing: an update. J Dermatol. 2001 Oct;28(10):521-34. Review.
2. Kossi J, Elenius K, Niinikoski J, Peltonen J, Laato M. Overview of wound healing. Ann Chir Gynaecol Suppl. 2001;(215):15-8. Review.

Infertility

Principles of Therapy:

Infertility is defined as the inability to conceive after 1 year of unprotected intercourse and affects approximately 10-15% of reproductive age couples. Most couples with infertility are sub-fertile, rather than absolutely infertile. Absolute infertility, meaning pregnancy rate of zero despite treatment, includes those individuals with bilateral tubal occlusion, amenorrhea secondary to gonadotropic cell destruction, ovarian or endometrial failure or absence of sperm. Only approximately 65% of infertility can be ascribed to the female. For female infertility, approximately 40% is related to ovulatory dysfunction, 40% to tubal and pelvic pathology and 10% due to anatomic disturbances or thyroid disease. Additionally, aging plays an important role in infertility and the risk of spontaneous abortion. Treatment protocols are generally aimed at alleviating the core etiology of infertility. This includes progestational agents for treating luteal phase defects, bromocriptine and other such agents for treating hyperprolactinemic conditions, and clomiphene citrate, GnRH, and other gonadotropins for treating ovulatory defects. Additionally, artifical reproductive techniques involving in vitro fertilization, intracytoplasmic sperm injection and donor egg programs are available. Ovulation induction frequently begins with clomiphene citrate which is an orally active medication which has a weak estrogenic effect and modifies the hypothalamic-pituitary axis so that response to estrogen levels is blunted and FSH and LH levels rise. Up to 80% of anovulatory women will ovulate with clomiphene and about 40% will conceive. Patients most likely to fail to ovulate with clomiphene include those with hyperandrogenism, polycystic ovaries, and obesity (insulin resistance). Weight loss plays an important role in the management of infertility in the obese patient. In patients with high androgen levels that fail to respond to clomiphene, the addition of dexamethasone improves ovulation and pregnancy rates. The induction of ovulation with human gonadotropins requires experience and careful patient evaluation as expense and side effects (both frequency and severity) are more common. Various products ranging from human menopausal gonadotropins collected from post-menopausal women to recombinate and purified products are now available. Gonadotropins are inactive orally and require intramuscular injection or subcutaneous administration. Human chorionic gonadotropin (HCG) may be used to simulate the mid-cycle LH surge during therapy to induce ovulation. Bromocriptine is also used in the treatment of infertile women with hyperprolactinemia and occasionally in those without elevated prolactin levels to improve responsiveness to clomiphene. This treatment in the lactating woman would not be advised as it would suppress prolactin production. Diagnosis of hyperprolactinemia would require a preexisting diagnosis as testing during lactation would produce altered results. Metformin also plays a role in the infertility treatment of women with polycystic ovaries and insulin resistance. While the complete therapy of infertility is beyond the scope of this test, several questions are pertinent to breastfeeding women. One, do these agents suppress lactation, or transfer into human milk and affect the infant? Secondly, does continued lactation and its coincident amenorrheic state reduce the fertility of the patient? In other words, should an infertile woman continue to breastfeed? The answers to these questions are not known for certain. Each of the agents commonly used in infertility will be described below.

BROMOCRIPTINE   AAP: Not Reviewed
Trade: Parlodel
Can/Aus/UK: Apo-Bromocriptine, Bromolactin, Kripton, Parlodel
Specifics: Bromocriptine is an anti-parkinsonian, synthetic ergot alkaloid which inhibits prolactin secretion. Maternal serum prolactin levels remain suppressed for up to 14 hours after a single dose. The FDA approved indication for lactation suppression has been withdrawn, and it is no longer approved for this purpose due to numerous maternal deaths, seizures, and strokes. It is sometimes used in hyperprolactinemic patients who have continued to breastfeed, although the incidence of maternal side-effects is significant and newer products are preferred. In one breastfeeding patient who received 5 mg/day for a pituitary tumor and continued breastfeeding, no untoward effects were noted in her infant. Caution is recommended as profound postpartum hypotension has been reported.
T1/2= 50 hours   Oral= <28%   Peak= 1-3 hours
LRC= L5

CABERGOLINE   AAP: Not Reviewed
Trade: Dostinex
Can/Aus/UK: Dostinex
Specifics: Cabergoline is a long-acting synthetic ergot alkaloid derivative which produces a dopamine agonist effect similar but much safer than bromocriptine (Parlodel). Cabergoline directly inhibits prolactin secretion by the pituitary. It is primarily indicated for pathological hyperprolactinemia, but in several European studies, it has been used for inhibition of post-partum lactation. In several European countries, cabergoline is indicated for the inhibition or suppression of physiologic lactation. The dose regimen used for the inhibition of physiologic lactation is cabergoline 1 mg administered as a single dose on the first day post-partum. For the suppression of established lactation, cabergoline 0.25 mg is taken every 12 hours for 2 days for a total of 1 mg. Single doses of 1 mg have been found to completely inhibit postpartum lactation. Transfer into human milk is not reported.
T1/2= 80 hours   Oral= Complete   Peak= 2-3 hours
LRC= L4

CLOMIPHENE CITRATE   AAP: Not Reviewed
Trade: Clomid, Serophene, Milophene
Can/Aus/UK: Clomid, Serophene
Specifics: In a study of 60 postpartum women (1-4 days postpartum), clomiphene was effective in totally inhibiting unestablished lactation, and in suppressing established lactation (day 4). It is not known if the use of clomiphene later postpartum affects milk production but it is unlikely and has not occurred in several cases of long-term lactation. Its transfer to the infant is unknown.
T1/2= 5-7 days   Oral= Complete   Peak= N/A
LRC= L4

DEXAMETHASONE   AAP: Not Reviewed
Trade: Decadron, Ak-dex, Maxidex
Can/Aus/UK: AK-Dex
Specifics: Dexamethasone is a long-acting corticosteroid, similar in effect to prednisone, although more potent. While the elimination half-life is brief, only 3-6 hours in adults, its metabolic effects last for up to 72 hours. No data are available on the transfer of dexamethasone into human milk. It is likely similar to that of prednisone which is extremely low. Doses of prednisone as high as 120 mg fail to produce clinically relevant milk levels. This product is commonly used in pediatrics for treating immune syndromes such as arthritis, and particularly acute onset asthma or other broncho constrictive diseases. It is not likely that the amount in milk would produce clinical effects unless used in high doses over prolonged periods.
T1/2= 3.3 hours   Oral= 78%   Peak= 1-2 hours
LRC= L3

GONADORELIN ACETATE   AAP: Not Reviewed
Trade: Lutrepulse
Can/Aus/UK: Lutrepulse, Wyeth-Ayerst HRF, Fertiral
Specifics: Gonadorelin has been detected in human breastmilk at concentrations of 0.1 to 3 nanogram/mL (adult dose = 20-100 micrograms) although its oral bioavailability in the infant would be minimal to none.
T1/2= 2-4 minutes   Oral= None   Peak= N/A
LRC= L3

HUMAN CHORIONIC GONADOTROPIN   AAP: Not Reviewed
Trade: Pregnyl, Profasi, A.P.L., Ovidrel
Can/Aus/UK: Pregnyl, Profasi
Specifics: Human chorionic gonadotropin (HCG) is a large polypeptide hormone produced by the human placenta with functions similar to luteinizing hormone (LH). Its function is to stimulate the corpus luteum of the ovary to produce progesterone, thus sustaining pregnancy. It is used for multiple purposes including pediatric

cryptorchidism, male hypogonadism, and ovulatory failure. HCG has no known effect on fat mobilization, appetite, sense of hunger or body fat distribution. HCG has NOT been found to be effective in treatment of obesity. Due to the large molecular weight (47,000) of HCG, it would be extremely unlikely penetrate into human milk. Further, it would not be orally bioavailable, due to destruction in the GI tract.

T1/2= 5.6 hours   Oral= 0%   Peak= 6 hours

MENOTROPINS   AAP: Not Reviewed
Trade: Pergonal, Humegon, Menogon
Can/Aus/UK: Pergonal, Humegon, Menogon
Specifics: Human Menopausal Gonadotropins are a purified mix of urinary gonadotropins from postmenopausal women containing FSH and LH activity. These are large molecular weight proteins and would not penetrate milk, nor likely suppress milk production. Purified and recombinant products are also available.

T1/2= 3.9 and 70.4 hours   Oral= 0%   Peak= 6 hours
LRC= L3

METFORMIN   AAP: Not Reviewed

Trade: Glucophage
Can/Aus/UK: Glucophage, Gen-Metformin, Glycon, Diabex, Diaformin, Diguanil
Specifics: In a preliminary study of 5 women who received 500 mg three times daily, milk levels were extremely low. While the average milk/plasma ratio was 0.34, the average dose to the infant was 0.0405 mg/kg/d or 0.26% of the weight-adjusted maternal dose. In this study, no adverse effects were noted in any infant.

T½= 6.2 hours(plasma)   Oral= 50%   Peak= 2.75 hours
LRC= L3

RECOMBINANT LH   AAP: Not Reviewed
Trade: LHadi
Can/Aus/UK:
Specifics: Recombinant Lutenizing hormone can also be used to simulate the midcycle LH surge.
T½= N/A   Oral= N/A   Peak= N/A
LRC= L3

Clinical Tips:
Progesterone is commonly used in some infertile patients to produce a secretory state of the endometrium. In most breastfeeding patients, excess progesterone has not been found to suppress lactation, nor penetrate to the infant in clinically relevant doses. Estrogens, however, particularly when used early postpartum can suppress lactation significantly and should be avoided if possible. In some patients,

clomiphene (Clomid, Serophene) is the first-line drug of choice for chronic anovulation, luteal phase defects, and unexplained infertility in patients with normal estrogen levels. When used early in lactation, clomiphene has been documented to completely suppress lactation. However, when used several months postpartum, it is believed to have minimal or no effect on milk production. Gonadorelin (Lutrepulse) is used for the induction of ovulation in anovulatory women with primary hypothalamic amenorrhea. Gonadorelin is a small decapeptide identical to the physiologic GnRH secreted by the hypothalamus which stimulates the pituitary release of luteinizing hormone (LH) and to a lesser degree follicle stimulating hormone (FSH). Gonadorelin has been detected in human breastmilk at concentrations of 0.1 to 3 nanogram/mL (adult dose = 20-100 micrograms), although its oral bioavailability in the infant would be minimal to none. Its ability to suppress lactation is unknown, but unlikely. Menotropins (Pergonal, Humegon) is a purified mix of urinary gonadotropins from postmenopausal women and produces FSH and LH activity. FSH and LH are large molecular weight proteins and would not penetrate milk, nor likely suppress milk production. In some infertile patients with hyperprolactinemia, bromocriptine, and more recently cabergoline (Dostinex) have been used to suppress plasma prolactin levels. These agents would be contraindicated in breastfeeding women, as they would dramatically suppress lactation.

Suggested Reading:

1. Carson DS, et al. Infertility in women: an update. J Am Pharm Assoc (Wash). 1998 Jul-Aug;38(4):480-6; quiz 487-8. Review.
2. Hanson MA, et al. Initial evaluation and treatment of infertility in a primary-care setting. Mayo Clin Proc. 1998 Jul;73(7):681-5. Review.
3. Hargreave TB, et al. Investigating and managing infertility in general practice. BMJ. 1998 May 9;316(7142):1438-41. Review.
4. Speroff L, Glass R, Kase N. Clinical Gynecologic Endocrinology and Infertility. Wolters Kluwer publishers. 6th edition, 1999.

Inflammatory Bowel Disease

Principles of Therapy:
The term 'chronic idiopathic inflammatory bowel disease' includes ulcerative colitis (UC) and Crohn's disease. Ulcerative colitis is a chronic, recurrent disease characterized by mucosal inflammation of the colon only. Ulcerative colitis invariably involves the rectum and proximately into part or all of the colon. Unlike UC, Crohn's disease is a chronic, recurrent transmural inflammatory condition involving any segment of the GI tract from the mouth to anus, the terminal ileum being the most common site. Although these syndromes vary significantly in their presentation, their pharmacotherapy is quite similar and includes the use of aminosalicylates(5-ASA), corticosteroids, immunosuppressants, antibiotics, antidiarrheals, and opioid analgesics.

AZATHIOPRINE   AAP: Not Reviewed

Trade: Imuran
Can/Aus/UK: Imuran, Thioprine
Specifics: Azathioprine is a powerful immunosuppressive agent that is metabolized to 6-Mercaptopurine (6-MP). In two mothers receiving 75 mg azathioprine, the concentration of 6-Mercaptopurine in milk varied from 3.5-4.5 µg/L in one mother, and 18 µg/L in the second mother. The authors conclude that these levels would be too low to produce clinical effects in a breastfed infant. Using this data for 6-MP, an infant would absorb only 0.1% of the weight-adjusted maternal dose which is too low to likely produce adverse effects in a breastfeeding infant. One infant continued to breastfeed during therapy and displayed no immunosuppressive effects.
T½= 0.6 hours   Oral= 41%   Peak= 1-2hours
LRC= L3

INFLIXIMAB   AAP: Not Reviewed

Trade: Remicade
Can/Aus/UK: Remicade
Specifics: Infliximab is a monoclonal antibody specific for tumor necrosis factor-alpha (TNF-alpha) and is used to treat Crohns disease and rheumatoid arthritis. Infliximab is a very large molecular weight antibody and is largely retained in the vascular system. In a study of one breastfeeding patient who received 5 mg/kg I.V., infliximab levels were determined in milk at 0, 2, 4, 8, 24, 48, 72 hours, and 4, 5, and 7 days. None was detected in milk at any time (detection limit < 0.1 µg/mL). While these are preliminary study results that are continuing, infliximab is probably too large to enter milk in clinically measurable amounts. It would not be orally bioavailable.

T½= 89.5 days LRC= L3   Oral= Nil   Peak= 1 hour

MESALAMINE
AAP: Give with caution

Trade: Asacol, Pentasa, Rowasa
Can/Aus/UK: Salofalk, Mesasal, Quintasa, Mesalazine, Asacol
Specifics: Mesalamine is 5-aminosalicylic acid and releases 5-ASA in the small bowel. Mesalamine is poorly absorbed from the GI tract. Only 5-35% of a dose is absorbed. In one patient receiving 500 mg mesalamine orally three times daily, the concentration of 5-ASA in breastmilk was 0.11 mg/L, and the Acetyl-5-ASA metabolite was 12.4 mg/L of milk. Using this data, the weight-adjusted relative infant dose would be 7.5% although most of this is not absorbed.
T½= 5-10 hours(metabolite)   Oral= 15-35%   Peak= 4-12 hours
LRC= L3

OLSALAZINE
AAP: Give with caution

Trade: Dipentum
Can/Aus/UK: Dipentum
Specifics: Olsalazine is bio-converted by colonic bacteria to 5-minosalicylic acid. Bioavailability is low and published milk levels are quite low.
T½= 0.9 hours   Oral= 2.4% (olsalazine)   Peak= 1-2 hours
LRC= L3

PREDNISONE
AAP: Compatible

Trade: Deltasone, Meticorten, Orasone
Can/Aus/UK: Apo-Prednisone, Deltasone, Novo-Prednisone, Sone, Panafcort, Decortisyl, Econosone
Specifics: The transfer of prednisone (PO) into milk is reported to be quite low. Doses as high as 120 mg daily do not produce clinically relevant doses via milk (47 µg/day).
T½= 3 hours(elimination)   Oral= 92%   Peak= 1-2 hours
LRC= L2
     L4 for chronic high doses

SULFASALAZINE
AAP: Give with caution

Trade: Azulfidine
Can/Aus/UK: PMS Sulfasalazine, Salazopyrin, SAS-500
Specifics: Sulfasalazine is bio-converted by colonic bacteria to 5-aminosalicylic acid and sulfapyridine. Most of the reported side effects are due to the sulfa component and are largely dose related. Bioavailability is low and published milk levels are quite low.

T½= 7.6 hours   Oral= Poor   Peak= Prolonged
LRC= L3

Clinical Tips:

Initial therapy of UC and Crohn's disease is with the 5-aminosalicylic acid products. Preparations of 5-ASA are formulated to release the drug at specific sites in the GI tract to intensify efficacy.   5-ASA is a topical agent that has a variety of anti-inflammatory effects. It is used during the active phase of inflammation and during disease inactivity to maintain remission. Sulfasalazine is bio-converted by bacterial azoreductases in the colon to 5-ASA and sulfapyridine. Olsalazine is converted to two molecules of 5-ASA. 5-ASA is virtually unabsorbed although high doses may induce (although remote) watery diarrhea in some breastfed infants.   Mesalamine (5-ASA) is primarily released in the small intestine, and is useful for Crohn's disease in that segment of the GI tract.   Prednisone, both oral and rectal, is a common component of therapy. Numerous studies show that oral prednisone penetrates milk poorly.   Rather high doses do not apparently produce significant levels in milk. However, some caution is due and close monitoring of the infant's growth rate is warranted.   With severe UC and Crohn's disease, immunosuppressants are warranted, particularly 6-MP.   It is not presently known if azathioprine or 6-MP penetrate milk but some transfer to the infant is likely.   The use of methotrexate in breastfeeding mothers is risky and questionable. Some studies question the efficacy of methotrexate in UC anyway. Methotrexate penetrates milk at low levels (2.6 µg/L) but its affinity for gastric mucosa in infants is high and concerning.   Recently, the use of the anti-TNF product infliximab(Remicade) has become popular. Infliximab is a large molecular weight protein and in one preliminary study by this author is not detectable in human milk following high IV doses. It would not likely be orally bioavailable anyway.   Further study is underway in other mothers but it appears safe for use in breastfeeding mothers.

Suggested Reading:

1.   Rutgeerts P. Medical therapy of inflammatory bowel disease.   Digestion. 1998 Aug;59(5):453-69. Review.
2.   Fiocchi C. Inflammatory bowel disease: etiology and pathogenesis. Gastroenterology. 1998 Jul;115(1):182-205. Review.
3.   Moses PL, et al. Inflammatory bowel disease. 1. Origins, presentation, and course. Postgrad Med. 1998 May;103(5):77-84. Review.
4.   Moses PL, et al. Inflammatory bowel disease. 2. Current and future therapeutic options. Postgrad Med. 1998 May;103(5):86-90, 95-7, 101-2. Review.
5.   Hale, TW. and Fasanmade, A. Unpublished data. 2002.

Insufficient Milk Supply

Principles of Therapy:

While insufficient milk production is one of the most commonly perceived dysfunctions in breastfeeding, it occurs rarely. Because new mothers often worry that the infant is receiving insufficient volumes of milk, this is almost universally the main reason that many new mothers give for early weaning and for supplementation with formulas. The vast majority of women who wean due to suspected poor supply are incorrect in their perception. Objective evidence for insufficient milk supply should be sought prior to beginning pharmacologic therapy. Further support for the social component regarding milk production is that several other cultures often complain of oversupply, rather than undersupply. Because it is difficult to ascertain how much volume the infant is receiving, even in infants that are gaining and thriving, the mother frequently worries that her supply is insufficient. Prior to assuming insufficient milk production, the clinician must assess a number of critical indicators such as: 1) number of stools per day (normally 5-10 by the end of the first week) but varies depending on age of the child, 2) the number of wet diapers per day (at least 6-8), 3) the baby should show no signs of dehydration or hyperbilirubinemia and 4) the infant is gaining weight along an acceptable growth curve. An insufficient milk supply may predispose to hyperbilirubinemia. The definitive indicator of sufficiency in the early neonatal period is infant weight gain. Specialized infant scales are available to allow pre and post feeding weights in an attempt to quantify the amount of milk received at a nursing.

METOCLOPRAMIDE   AAP: Compatible
    Trade: Reglan
    Can/Aus/UK: Apo-Metoclop, Emex, Maxeran, Reglan, Maxolon, Pramin, Gastromax, Paramid
    Specifics: Peak metoclopramide levels in milk occur at 2-3 hours after administration of the medication. During the late puerperium, the concentration of metoclopramide in the milk varied from 20 to 125µg/L, which was less than the 28 to 157µg/L noted during the early puerperium. The authors estimated the daily dose to infant to vary from 6 to 24µg/kg/day during the early puerperium, and from 1 to 13µg/kg/day during the late phase. These doses are minimal compared to those used for therapy of reflux in pediatric patients (0.1 to 0.5 mg/kg/day). In these studies, only 1 of 5 infants studied had detectable blood levels of metoclopramide, hence no accumulation or side effects were observed.
    T1/2= 5-6 hours   Oral= 30-100%   Peak= 1-2 hours
    LRC= L2

186

DOMPERIDONE   **AAP:** Compatible
Trade:
Can/Aus/UK: Motilium, Motilidone
Specifics: Domperidone blocks peripheral dopamine receptors in the GI
wall and in the CRTZ (nausea center) in the brain stem and is currently used
as an antiemetic.   Unlike metoclopramide, it does not enter the brain
compartment, and it has few CNS effects such as depression. It is also known
to produce significant increases in prolactin levels and has proven useful as a
galactagogue.   Concentrations of domperidone reported in milk vary
according to dose but following a dose of 10 mg three times daily, the average
concentration in milk was 2.6 µg/L.
T1/2= 7-14 hours   Oral= 13-17%   Peak= 30 minutes
LRC= L2

SULPIRIDE   **AAP:** Not Reviewed
Trade:
Can/Aus/UK: Dolmatil, Sulparex, Sulpitil
Specifics: In a study with 14 women who received sulpiride (50 mg three
times daily), and in a subsequent study with 36 breastfeeding women,
Ylikorkala found major increases in prolactin levels and significant, but only
moderate increases in breastmilk production.   In a group of 20 women who
received 50 mg twice daily, breastmilk samples were drawn 2 hours after the
dose.   The concentration of sulpiride in breastmilk ranged from 0.26 to
1.97µg/mL. No effects on breastfed infants were noted.
T1/2= 6-8 hours   Oral= 27-34 %   Peak= 2-6 hours
LRC= L2

Clinical Tips:

While extremely rare, some women may have true insufficient milk supply as a
function of a number of problems including: insufficient glandular tissue, breast
surgery or reduction, mammoplasty with severing of the ductal tissues near the
nipple, anemia, shock or postpartum hemorrhage. Placement of breast implants is of
minor concern for insufficient milk supply (3 fold increase) unless a peri-areolar
incision has been used. This type of incision involves severing of more ducts and
nerves to the areola and has been associated with a five fold increased incidence of
low milk supply. Breast reduction can be performed either by nipple translocation
(complete removal and reattachment of the nipple) or by using an inferior pedicle
technique. Even with the latter, there is a great deal of damage to the nerves and
ductal system. In any of these cases, mothers with breast surgeries should be advised
to notify the infant's care provider of their surgical history. Regardless of the cause
for low milk supply, continued frequent breastfeeding and if needed use of a tube-
feeding device to deliver added nutrient to the infant until supply increases is
indicated. Warm compresses applied to the breasts and relaxation techniques may be
of benefit. In those cases where engorgement occurs without letdown, then

intranasal oxytocin may be required. In patients with severe feeding problems, a certified lactation consultant should be consulted, and only then should one attempt to increase the supply with metoclopramide or domperidone. Metoclopramide has multiple functions but is primarily used for increasing the lower esophageal sphincter tone in gastroesophageal reflux in patients with reduced gastric tone. It is sometimes used in lactating women to stimulate prolactin release from the pituitary and enhance breastmilk production. Since 1981, a number of publications have documented major increases in breastmilk production following the use of metoclopramide, domperidone, or sulpiride.

With metoclopramide, the increase in serum prolactin and breastmilk production appears dose-related up to a dose of 15 mg three times daily. Many studies show 66 to 100% increases in milk production depending on the degree breastmilk supply in the mother prior to therapy. In another study of 23 women with premature infants, milk production increased from 93 mL/day to 197 mL/day between the 1st and 7th day of therapy with 30 mg/day. Prolactin levels, although varied, increased from 18.1 to 121.8 ng/mL. Gupta studied 32 mothers with inadequate milk supply. Following a dose of 10 mg three times daily, a 66-100% increase in milk supply was noted. No untoward effects were noted in the infants. Doses of 15 mg/day were found ineffective, whereas doses of 30-45 mg/day were most effective. In most studies, major increases in prolactin were observed, such as 18.1 ng/mL to 121.8 ng/mL after therapy in one study. While it is well recognized that metoclopramide increases milk supply, it is very dose-dependent and some mothers simply do not respond. Side effects such as gastric cramping and diarrhea limit the compliance of some patients. Further, it is often found that upon discontinuing the medication, the supply of milk reduces rapidly. A slow tapering of the dose over several weeks is generally recommended in those women who respond. Long-term use of this medication (>4 weeks) is not generally recommended as the incidence of depression increases. As post-partum depression carries a high likelihood of recurrence, use of metoclopramide in a mother with prior history of depression provides a relative contraindication. If metoclopramide fails to work within 7 days, it is unlikely that longer therapy will be effective.

Domperidone, due to minimal side effects and superior efficacy, is a better choice galactogogue but is unfortunately not available in the USA. Recently it has become available through compounding pharmacies with a prescription. The usual oral dose for controlling GI distress is 10-20 mg three to four times daily although for nausea and vomiting the dose can be higher(up to 40 mg). The galactagogue dose is suggested to be 10-20 mg orally 3-4 times daily. Sulpiride is a selective dopamine antagonist used as an antidepressant and antipsychotic. Several studies using smaller doses have found it to significantly increase prolactin levels and breastmilk production in smaller doses that do not produce overt neuroleptic effects on the mother.

Multiple herbal therapies are touted as benefiting poor milk supply. Scientific evidence supporting the effectiveness of many of these compounds is limited. Concern also exists regarding the relative potency and quality control of herbal products in the United States. Fenugreek in doses of 3 tablets three times daily has been suggested to improve milk supply. In a case-control study of 10 exclusively breast pumping women, the increase in milk production was > 20% in 5 of 10 mothers and >100% in 3 of these. Further study is needed regarding the safety and effectiveness of herbal galactogogues.

Suggested Reading:

1. Kauppila A. et.al. A dose response relation between improved lactation and metoclopramide. The Lancet 1:1175-77, 1981.
2. Budd SC. et.al. Improved lactation with metoclopramide. Clinical Pediatrics 32:53-57, 1993.
3. Kauppila A, et.al. Metoclopramide and Breast Feeding: Transfer into milk and the newborn. Eur. J. Clin Pharmacol. 25:819-23, 1983.
4. Ehrenkranz RA. et.al. Metoclopramide effect on faltering milk production by mothers of premature infants. Pediatrics 78:614-620, 1986.
5. Gupta AP and Gupta PK. Metoclopramide as a lactagogue. Clinical Pediatrics 24:269-72, 1985.
6. Hofmeyr GJ and van Iddekinge B. Domperidone and lactation. Lanet i, 647, 1983.
7. Hofmeyr GJ, et.al. Domperidone: secretion in breastmilk and effect on puerperal prolactin levels. Brit. J. Obs. and Gyn. 92:141-144, 1985.
8. Wiesel FA, Alfredsson G, Ehrnebo M et al: The pharmacokinetics of intravenous and oral sulpiride in healthy human subjects. Eur J Clin Pharmacol 17:385-391, 1980.
9. Ylikorkala O, Kauppila A, Kivinen S et al: Sulpiride improves inadequate lactation. Br Med J 285:249-251, 1982.
10. Ylikorkala O, Kauppila A, Kivinen S et al: Treatment of inadequate lactation with oral sulpiride and buccal oxytocin. Obstet Gynecol 1984; 63:57-60.
11. Aono T, Shioji T, et.al. Augmentation of puerperal lactation by oral administration of sulpiride. J. Clin. Endo. Metabol. 48(3): 478-482, 1979.

Low Back Pain

Principles of Therapy:

Low back pain is exceedingly common, occurring in over 80% of the population. The differential diagnosis is broad and includes disk herniation, degenerative arthritis, and metastatic cancer. Among the many suffers of low back pain, the diagnostic challenge is to discern those few patients who require additional diagnostic work up. In principle this means identifying those patients whose pain is due to infection, carcinoma, inflammatory back disease, disk herniation, spondylitic syndromes, and leaking aortic aneurysm. Most back pain resolves within several weeks to one month and early mobilization is generally recommended following the acute attack. Pharmacotherapy is only marginally effective in many of these syndromes and is comprised primarily of nonsteroidal anti-inflammatory medications, steroid injections, and opioids in some patients. A newer therapy using the anticonvulsants, particularly gabapentin, is proving significantly effective in some patients.

ACETAMINOPHEN   **AAP**: Compatible

Trade: Tempra, Tylenol, Paracetamol
Can/Aus/UK: Apo-Acetaminophen, Tempra, Tylenol, Paracetamol, Panadol, Dymadon, Calpol
Specifics: Only minimal amounts are secreted in milk.
T½= 2 hours   Oral= >85%   Peak= 0.5-2 hours
LRC= L1

AMITRIPTYLINE   **AAP**: May be of
                                                            concern
Trade: Elavil, Endep
Can/Aus/UK: Apo-Amitriptyline, Elavil, Novo-Tryptin, Amitrol, Endep, Mutabon D, Tryptanol, Domical, Lentizol
Specifics: Levels in breastmilk are reported to be quite small. Numerous studies indicate minimal effects on nursing infant.
T½= 31-46 hours   Oral= Complete   Peak= 2-4 hours
LRC= L2

CODEINE   **AAP**: Compatible

Trade: Empirin #3 # 4, Tylenol # 3 # 4
Can/Aus/UK: Paveral, Penntuss, Actacode, Codalgin, Codral, Panadeine, Veganin, Kaodene, Teropin
Specifics: Breastmilk levels of codeine are minimal, if the dose is kept less than 60 mg.

T½= 2.9 hours   Oral= Complete   Peak= 0.5-1 hr.
LRC= L3

HYDROCODONE   AAP: Not Reviewed

Trade: Lortab, Vicodin
Can/Aus/UK:
Specifics: Although we have minimal data on hydrocodone's transfer to milk, its use in breastfeeding women is widespread and only occasional sedation has been reported.
T½= 3.8 hours   Oral= Complete   Peak= 1.3 hours
LRC= L3

IBUPROFEN   AAP: Compatible

Trade: Advil, Nuprin, Motrin, Pediaprofen
Can/Aus/UK: Actiprofen, Advil, Amersol, Motrin, ACT-3, Brufen, Nurofen, Rafen
Specifics: Ibuprofen is an ideal NSAID for breastfeeding mother due to short half-life and minimal breastmilk levels.
T½= 1.8-2.5 hours   Oral= 80%   Peak= 1-2 hours
LRC= L1

IMIPRAMINE   AAP: May be of
                                                        concern

Trade: Tofranil, Janimine
Can/Aus/UK: Apo-Imipramine, Impril, Novo-Pramine, Melipramine, Tofranil
Specifics: Dose via milk is low and is estimated to be from 20-200 ug per day. No untoward effects noted in breastfed infants.
T½= 8-16 hours   Oral= 90%   Peak= 1-2 hours
LRC= L2

METAXALONE   AAP: Not Reviewed

Trade: Skelaxin
Can/Aus/UK:
Specifics: While we have no breastfeeding data with this product, it produces a low degree of sedation and other major side effects and could possibly be used briefly in breastfeeding mothers.
T½= 2-3 hours   Oral= N/A   Peak= 2 hours
LRC= L3

NAPROXEN   AAP: Compatible

Trade: Anaprox, Naprosyn, Naproxen, Aleve
Can/Aus/UK: Anaprox, Apo-Naproxen, Naprosyn, Naxen, Inza, Proxen SR, Synflex
Specifics: Naproxen is a longer half-life NSAID and as such is should not be used for long periods in order to prevent buildup in the infant. Infrequent use is not contraindicated, particularly with older infants.
T½= 12-15 hours   Oral= 74-99%   Peak= 2-4 hours
LRC= L3
          L4 for chronic use

GABAPENTIN   AAP: Not Reviewed

Trade: Neurontin
Can/Aus/UK: Neurontin
Specifics: No published data are available on this drug, but its lack of significant sedation may suggest it suitable for breastfeeding women. However, in preliminary results from two patients studied in our own laboratories indicate a modest infant dose via milk. In one breastfeeding mother who was receiving 1800 mg/d, milk levels were 11.1, 11.1, 11.3, and 11.0 mg/L at 0, 2, 4, and 8 hours, respectively, following a dose of 600 mg. The maternal and infant plasma levels at 2 hours post dose were 16.6 mg/L and less than 0.3 mg/L respectively. In another mother receiving 2400 mg/d milk levels were 4.6, 9.8, 9.0, and 7.2 mg/L at 0, 2, 4, and 8 hours respectively, after a dose of 800 mg. The maternal plasma level at 2 hours post dose was 15.1 mg/L. Using these limited data, the calculated relative infant doses were approximately 6.0% to 3.1% respectively, of the weight-adjusted maternal dose. No adverse events were noted in either of these two infants.
T½= 5-7 hours   Oral= 50-60%   Peak= 1-3 hours
LRC= L3

Clinical Tips:
Treatment of low back pain is generally palliative at best. For the most part, the NSAIDs are poorly effective but may be used briefly. Ibuprofen should be preferred, as milk levels are negligible. Naproxen could be used briefly. The use of the tricyclics antidepressants for chronic pain is well documented. Amitriptyline and imipramine have been well studied in breastfeeding women and appear safe in most instances. New studies have shown that the newer anticonvulsants such as gabapentin are significantly effective in chronic low back pain and radiculopathy. Although any of the anticonvulsants may be used, such as valproic acid or carbamazepine, the minimal side effect profile of gabapentin makes it a favorite with patients. Although we have limited data on gabapentin use in breastfeeding

mothers, its relative safety in humans is encouraging. While skeletal muscle relaxants have been used extensively, most studies find them minimally effective. Codeine and hydrocodone can be used in some patients in acute pain. Long term therapy is not advised.

Suggested Reading:

1. Goldsmith ME, et al. Clinical evaluation of low back pain. Compr Ther. 1998 Aug;24(8):370-7. Review.
2. Borenstein D. Epidemiology, etiology, diagnostic evaluation, and treatment of low back pain. Curr Opin Rheumatol. 1998 Mar;10(2):104-9. Review.
3. Borenstein DG. A clinician's approach to acute low back pain. Am J Med. 1997 Jan 27;102(1A):16S-22S. Review.
4. Deyo RA, et al. Low back pain. A primary care challenge. Spine. 1996 Dec 15;21(24):2826-32. Review.
5. Hale TW, Ilett KF, Hackett P. Personnal communication, 2002.

Mastitis

Principles of Therapy:

Mastitis is a common and debilitating condition most often found in lactating women. It occurs most commonly in primigravida rather than multipara women. Both inflammatory and infectious mastitis have been described, but it is often difficult to differentiate. Most cases are considered infectious and are treated with antibiotic therapy with more often and complete emptying of the breast. The reported incidence varies, but approximately 20% of lactating women in the first 6 months postpartum will experience mastitis with the highest incidence 2-3 weeks postpartum. Mastitis most likely occurs as a result of introduction of organisms from the infants mouth and nostrils into an injured nipple. *Staphylococcus aureus* (occasionally penicillin resistant), *streptococcus*, and to a lesser degree *Escherichia coli* are the primary pathogens. Culture of breastmilk in routine circumstances is probably unwarranted but certan circumstances may indicate otherwise such as recurrent or persistent infections. Purported predisposing factors include; stress, fatigue, anemia, prior breast surgery, improper fitting bras, poor emptying of the breast, missed feeding with engorgement, overabundant milk supply, too frequent or infrequent feeds, cracked or damaged nipples, and plugged ducts. A recent study of mastitis occurring in 946 breastfeeding women found an incidence of 9.5% in the first 3 months post-partum. In this particular, study factors associated with mastitis include a history of mastitis with a prior infant, cracks and sore nipple within the preceding week, using anti-fungal cream within the preceding three weeks and using a manual breast pump. Discomfort for the mother can range from mild tenderness, to severe breast pain with fever, chills, malaise, flu-like symptoms, and myalgias. Wedge-shaped areas of the breast will appear pink, hot, swollen, and extremely tender. Breast abscess occurs in 5-10% of cases of mastitis and may be associated with delayed or inadequate treatment of mastitis. Treatment of mastitis includes antibiotics, rest, frequent milk removal, and pain control, often with an anti-inflammatory medication such as ibuprofen. Most authorities recommend antibiotic treatment for 10 to 14 days. There is no evidence that continued breastfeeding is harmful to the nursing infant and weaning during this time should be discouraged due to the potential increased risk for abscess formation.

CEFAZOLIN   AAP: Approved
   Trade: Ancef, Kefzol
   Can/Aus/UK: Ancef, Kefzol, Cefamezin
   Specifics: In 20 patients who received a 2 gm STAT dose over 10 minutes, the average   concentration of cefazolin in milk in 2, 3, and 4 hours after the dose was 1.25, 1.51, and 1.16 mg/L, respectively.
   T1/2= 1.2-2.2 hours   Oral= Poor   Peak= 1-2 hours
   LRC= L1

CEPHALEXIN   AAP: Approved
   Trade: Keflex
   Can/Aus/UK: Apo-Cephalex, Ceporex, Novo-Lexin, Ibilex, Keflex
   Specifics: Following a 1000 mg maternal oral dose, milk levels at 1, 2, 3, 4, and 5 hours ranged from 0.20, 0.28, 0.39, 0.50, and 0.47 mg/L respectively. Milk/serum ratios varied from 0.008 at 1 hour, to 0.140 at 3 hours. These levels are probably too low to be clinically relevant.
   T1/2= 50-80 minutes   Oral= Complete   Peak= 1 hour
   LRC= L1

CLINDAMYCIN   AAP: Approved
   Trade: Cleocin
   Can/Aus/UK: Dalacin, Clindatech, Cleocin
   Specifics: Following oral doses of 300 mg every 6 hours, the breastmilk levels averaged 1.0 to 1.7 mg/L at 1.5 to 7 hours after dosing. One case of pseudomembranous colitis has been reported following high-dose IV therapy.
   T1/2= 2.9 hours   Oral= 90%   Peak=45-60min (oral)
   LRC= L3

CLOXACILLIN   AAP: Not Reviewed
   Trade: Tegopen, Cloxapen
   Can/Aus/UK: Apo-Cloxi, Novo-Cloxin, Orbenin, Alclox, Kloxerate-DC
   Specifics: Following a single 500 mg oral dose of cloxacillin in lactating women, milk concentrations of the drug were zero to 0.2 mg/L one and two hours after the dose respectively, and 0.2 to 0.4 mg/L after 6 hours.
   T1/2= 0.7-3 hours   Oral= 37-60%   Peak= 0.5-2 hours
   LRC= L2

DICLOXACILLIN   AAP: Not Reviewed
   Trade: Pathocil, Dycill, Dynapen
   Can/Aus/UK: Diclocil
   Specifics: Following oral administration of a 250 mg dose, milk concentrations of the drug were 0.1, and 0.3 mg/L at 2 and 4 hours after the dose, respectively. Levels were undetectable after 6 hours.
   T1/2= 0.6-0.8 hours   Oral= 35-76%   Peak= 0.5-2 hours
   LRC= L1

FLOXACILLIN   AAP: Not Reviewed
   Trade: Flucil
   Can/Aus/UK: Flopen, Floxapen, Flu Clomix, Flu-Amp, Fluclox, Flucloxacillin, Magnapen, Staphylex
   Specifics: Floxacillin, also called flucloxacillin, is a penicillinase-resistant penicillin frequently used for resistant staphylococcal infections. Only trace amounts are secreted into human milk. Its congener cloxacillin, is commonly

195

used to treat mastitis in breastfeeding mothers and has been used in thousands of breastfeeding patients without problem. Changes in gut flora are possible but unlikely.

T1/2= 1.5 hours   Oral= 50%   Peak= 1 hour
LRC= L1

NAFCILLIN   AAP: Not Reviewed
Trade: Unipen, Nafcil
Can/Aus/UK: Unipen
Specifics: No data are available on the concentration of nafcillin in milk, but it is likely small. Oral absorption in the infant would be minimal.
T1/2= 0.5-1.5 hours   Oral= 50%   Peak= 30-60 min(IM)
LRC= L1

VANCOMYCIN   AAP: Not Reviewed
Trade: Vancocin
Can/Aus/UK: Vancocin, Vancoled
Specifics: Milk levels were 12.7 mg/L four hours after infusion in one woman receiving 1 gm every 12 hours for 7 days. Its poor absorption from the infant's GI tract would limit its systemic absorption.
T1/2= 5.6 hours   Oral= Minimal   Peak= N/A
LRC= L1

Clinical Tips:
Management of lactational mastitis includes the use of antibiotics when appropriate and effective draining of the breast. Most protocols suggest that the mother should continue to breastfeed on both breasts. Complete emptying of each breast is important, so occasional pumping may be required. Patients should be encouraged to reduce stress, use maternity bras (or none at all), rather than restrictive ill-fitting bras. The physician should insist on increased rest with frequent breastfeeding. Antibiotic therapy, particularly that which covers resistant Staph aureus, is now required. The clinician is urged to review sensitivities of staph organisms for their individual regions. Orally, in most individuals, dicloxacillin or cloxacillin are still quite effective at doses of 500 mg four times daily for 10-14 days and should be the first-line drugs of choice. Shorter courses are prone to relapse though controlled studies have not been done evaluating optimal length of treatment. Cephalexin is a good second-line drug of choice. Amoxicillin with clavulanate (Augmentin) is a third-line choice, but sensitivities may be useful prior to use. In individuals with penicillin hypersensitivities, cephalexin or clindamycin may be preferred. In individuals hypersensitive to cephalosporins and penicillins, erythromycin may be used if the organism is sensitive. In those individuals with severe infections, nafcillin IV, cefazolin IV, or clindamycin IV have been efficacious. When using nafcillin IV, the addition of 3-5 days of gentamicin (2-5 mg/kg/day) greatly stimulates synergism and increases efficacy. In extremely resistant Staph infections,

vancomycin IV is the drug of choice. New data suggests that adding rifampin will greatly reduce emergence of resistance. While erythromycin, other macrolide antibiotics, and sulfonamides have been useful in the past, the high degree of resistance to these agents may preclude their use today. Use of an anti-inflammatory medication such as ibuprofen is recommended for initial treatment of mastitis. This provides pain relief and the anti-inflammatory properties may assist with resolution of the inflammation during the early therapy of this infection. In patients with severe abscess, surgical drainage is required along with appropriate antibiotic therapy. Drainage may be accomplished by ultrasound guided needle aspiration or by traditional incision and drainage. Milk fistula is a rare (approximately 10%) complication of drainage of breast abscesses. This is a self limited condition and reassurance and techniques to contain the milk drainage should be offered. Needle aspiration of breast abscesses may result in a more pleasing cosmetic result than incision.

Suggested Reading:

1. Lawrence RA. In: Breastfeeding, a guide for the medical profession. Fourth Edition. Mosby, St. Louis. 1994.
2. Pernoll ML. In Current Obstetric and Gynecologic Diagnosis and Treatment. Seventh Edition, Appleton and Lange, Norwalk, CN.
3. Fetherston, C. Risk factors for lactation mastitis. J. Hum. Lact 14(2):101-109, 1998.
4. Bedinghaus JM. Care of the breast and support of breast-feeding. Prim.Care 24(1):147-60, 1997.
5. Schentag JJ, Hyatt JM, et.al. Genesis of Methicillin-resistant Staphylococcus aureus (MRSA), How treatment of MRSA infections has selected for Vancomycin-Resistant Enterococcus faecium, and the importance of antibiotic-management and infection control. Clin. Infect. Dis. 26:1204-14, 1998.

Metabolic Bone Disease

Principles of Therapy:

Metabolic bone disease denotes a number of conditions producing diffusely decreased bone density (osteopenia) and reduced bone strength. Histologically it is characterized as: osteoporosis (reduced bone matrix and decreased mineral content) and osteomalacia (bone matrix intact and decreased mineral content). Osteoporosis is the most common bone disease in the USA and accounts for thousands of bone fractures annually. Interestingly, in osteoporosis the rate of bone production is normal, while the rate of bone resorption is significantly elevated. Osteomalacia is generally a result of poor mineralization of the bone, simply put, a result of poor calcium intake. In children this is called rickets, while in adults it is called osteomalacia. Treatment of these two syndromes largely depends on the etiology. In postmenopausal women, estrogen replacement is generally recommended in suitable cases. While calcium and phosphate replacement help, they only slow bone loss, they do not necessarily replace lost bone density. The chronic use of high dose steroids also predisposes to osteoporosis. The use of the medications below first require accurate diagnosis of the etiology of the syndrome prior to use.

ESTROGEN-ESTRADIOL   AAP: Compatible

Trade: Estratab, Premarin, Menest
Can/Aus/UK:
Specifics: Estrogens enter milk in minimal quantities, however they may suppress milk production during lactation.
T½= 60 minutes   Oral= Complete   Peak= Rapid
LRC= L3

FLUORIDE   AAP: Approved

Trade: Pediaflor, Flura
Can/Aus/UK:
Specifics: Fluoride is present in milk at rather low levels (< 0.172 ppm) in a normal population with 0.7 ppm in drinking water. Fluoride probably forms calcium fluoride salts in milk that may limit the oral bioavailability of the fluoride provided by human milk. Maternal supplementation is unnecessary and not recommended in areas with high fluoride content (> 0.7 ppm) in water. Allergy to fluoride has been reported in one infant. The American Academy of Pediatrics no longer recommends supplementing of breastfed infants with oral fluoride.
T½= 6 hours   Oral= 90%   Peak= N/A
LRC= L2

VITAMIN D

AAP: Compatible

Trade: Calciferol, Delta-D, Vitamin D
Can/Aus/UK:
Specifics: Vitamin D content in milk is rather low, but milk levels are proportional to maternal serum levels and maternal intake. Adequate daily intake is recommended but supra therapeutic doses are not advised.
T½= N/A   Oral= Variable   Peak= N/A
LRC= L3

ALENDRONATE SODIUM

AAP: Not Reviewed

Trade: Fosamax
Can/Aus/UK: Fosamax
Specifics: Maternal plasma levels of alendronate are barely detectable, thus milk levels would probably be undetectable. Extremely poor oral bioavailability would severely limit oral absorption from milk.
T½= <3 hours(plasma)   Oral= <0.7%   Peak= N/A
LRC= L3

ETIDRONATE

AAP: Not Reviewed

Trade: Didronel
Can/Aus/UK: Didronel
Specifics: Maternal plasma levels of etidronate are barely detectable, thus milk levels would probably be undetectable. Extremely poor oral bioavailability would severely limit oral absorption from milk.
T½= 6 hours(plasma)   Oral= 1-2.5%   Peak= 2 hours
LRC= L3

CALCITONIN

AAP: Not Reviewed

Trade: Calcimar, Salmonine, Osteocalcin, Miacalcin
Can/Aus/UK: Caltine, Calcimar, Calcitare, Calsynar, Miacalcic
Specifics: The large molecular weight of this compound would preclude its entry into milk. Further, calcitonin oral bioavailability is nil.
T½= 1 hour   Oral= None   Peak= 2 hours
LRC= L3

Clinical Tips:

Calcitonin is a large molecular weight protein and is unlikely to penetrate milk to any degree. It is not orally bioavailable. Estrogen replacement therapy in postmenopausal, or hypogonadal women, is known to reduce bone loss but does not increase bone density to any degree. Unfortunately, the use of estrogen in breastfeeding women carries a high risk of significantly suppressing breastmilk production, particularly during the first 4-6 months postpartum and somewhat less thereafter. Studies suggest that with higher calcium doses, estrogen doses can be reduced. Vitamin D is an oil soluble vitamin. Although we do not know how much transfers into milk, milk levels are apparently in equilibrium with the maternal plasma. Thus high maternal doses should be used with caution in breastfeeding mothers. The biphosphonates (e.g. alendronate, etidronate) inhibit osteoclast mediated bone resorption by depositing in bone for long periods. Potential side effects of bisphosphonate therapy may include bone pain, gastritis, esophagitis, and possible bone marrow abnormalities. Due to their plasma kinetics and poor oral bioavailability, they are not likely to induce problems in breastfed infants, but we have no data showing safety as of yet. Fluoride decreases bone turnover and has occasionally been used in osteoporotic patients. While it appears efficacious in improving bone mineral density there is concern that it may be ineffective in fracture provention. While its transfer in milk is modest to low, the use of large doses of fluoride in breastfeeding mothers is unwise. Side effects in adult patients on high doses of fluoride are significant, and interestingly, although the bone density increased, the bone strength did not. Lower doses (30-50 mg) are now in vogue. These doses are still far too high for breastfeeding mothers.

Suggested Reading:

1. Andrews WC. What's new in preventing and treating osteoporosis? Postgrad Med. 1998 Oct;104(4):89-92, 95-7. Review.
2. Lenchik L, et al. Orthopedic aspects of metabolic bone disease. Orthop Clin North Am. 1998 Jan;29(1):103-34. Review.
3. Metabolic bone disease. Curr Opin Rheumatol. 1997 Jul;9(4):B142-57.

Migraine Headache

Principles of Therapy:

Classic migraine headache is a lateralized throbbing headache that occurs episodically. The symptoms of migraine vary enormously between patients, and the classification is largely based on the headache's characteristics and associated symptoms. Two major varieties of migraine have been described and are the migraine with aura (classic migraine) or the migraine without aura (common migraine). The aura is a focal neurologic symptom that often precedes the attack, and may consist of visual hallucinations such as stars, sparks, light flashes, and luminous hallucinations (scintillating scotomas). The etiology of migraine is obscure, but may be a genetically transmitted functional disturbance of intracranial circulation. Migraine attacks are believed to be preceded by an intense regional vasoconstriction. The relative ischemia and subsequent release of local cytokines may induce the aura in some patients. The ischemic phase is subsequently followed by an intense vasodilation, which is generally associated with pain. Nausea occurs in 90% of patients as well as photophobia, phonophobia, and blurred vision. Treatment of migraine is either to prevent the acute episode or to prevent future attacks (prophylactic). Acute therapies include mild opioids, ergot alkaloids, antiemetics, sedatives, caffeine adjuvant compound, and serotonin agonists. Prophylactic therapies include beta-blockers, calcium channel blockers, antidepressants, serotonin antagonists, and anticonvulsants. In patients with mild to moderate pain, therapy includes the use of analgesics, acetaminophen, mild sedatives, or NSAIDs. If treatment fails, sumatriptan or transnasal butorphanol may be required. Ergot alkaloids should be absolutely avoided in breastfeeding mothers during the first 6 months postpartum and during pregnancy.

ACETAMINOPHEN
AAP: Compatible

Trade: Tempra, Tylenol, Paracetamol
Can/Aus/UK: Apo-Acetaminophen, Tempra, Tylenol, Paracetamol, Panadol, Dymadon, Calpol
Specifics: Only minimal amounts are secreted in milk.
T½= 2 hours   Oral= >85%   Peak= 0.5-2 hours
LRC= L1

AMITRIPTYLINE
AAP: May be of concern

Trade: Elavil, Endep
Can/Aus/UK: Apo-Amitriptyline, Elavil, Novo-Tryptin, Amitrol, Endep,Mutabon D, Tryptanol, Domical, Lentizol
Specifics: Levels in breastmilk are reported to be quite small. Numerous

studies indicate minimal effects on nursing infant.

T½= 31-46 hours　　　Oral= Complete　　　Peak= 2-4 hours
LRC= L2

BUTALBITOL COMPOUND　　　　　　　　AAP: Not Reviewed

Trade:　Fioricet, Fiorinal, Bancap, Two-dyne
Can/Aus/UK:
Specifics:　No data are available on transfer into milk.　Butalbitol is a barbiturate. Occasional use is unlikely to sedate an infant.
T½= 40-140 hours　　　Oral= Complete　　　Peak= 40-60 min.
LRC= L3

BUTORPHANOL　　　　　　　　　　　　AAP: Compatible

Trade:　Stadol
Can/Aus/UK:
Specifics:　Milk levels are extremely low (< 4 µg/L).
T½= 3-4 hours　　　　Oral= 17 %　　　　Peak= 1 hour
LRC= L3

CODEINE　　　　　　　　　　　　　　AAP: Compatible

Trade:　Empirin #3 # 4, Tylenol # 3 # 4
Can/Aus/UK:　Paveral, Penntuss, Actacode, Codalgin, Codral, Panadeine, Veganin, Kaodene, Teropin
Specifics:　Breastmilk levels of codeine are minimal, if the dose is kept less than 60 mg.
T½= 2.9 hours　　　　Oral= Complete　　　Peak= 0.5-1 hr.
LRC= L3

IBUPROFEN　　　　　　　　　　　　　AAP: Compatible

Trade:　Advil, Nuprin, Motrin, Pediaprofen
Can/Aus/UK:　Actiprofen, Advil, Amersol, Motrin, ACT-3, Brufen, Nurofen, Rafen
Specifics:　Ibuprofen is an ideal NSAID for breastfeeding mothers due to short half-life and minimal breastmilk levels.
T½= 1.8-2.5 hours　　　Oral= 80%　　　Peak= 1-2 hours
LRC= L1

KETOROLAC

AAP: Compatible

Trade: Toradol, Acular
Can/Aus/UK: Acular, Toradol
Specifics: In a study of 10 patients receiving 10 mg PO four times daily ketorolac was undetectable in 4 milk samples and exceedingly low in the other 6 patient samples (5.2-7.3 µg/L). While the manufacturer does not approve use in breastfeeding mothers, the levels in breastmilk are incredibly low, far too low to induce clinical effects in a breastfeeding infant.   No evidence of untoward effects in infants has been published.
T½= 2.4-8.6 hours   Oral= >81%   Peak= 0.5 - 1 hr.
LRC= L2

METOCLOPRAMIDE

AAP: Compatible

Trade: Reglan
Can/Aus/UK: Apo-Metoclop, Emex, Maxeran, Reglan, Maxolon, Pramin, Gastromax, Paramid
Specifics: Peak metoclopramide levels in milk occur at 2-3 hours after administration of the medication.   During the late puerperium,   the concentration of metoclopramide in the milk varied from 20 to 125µg/L, which was less than the 28 to 157µg/L noted during the early puerperium. The authors estimated the daily dose to infant to vary from 6 to 24µg/kg/day during the early puerperium, and from 1 to 13µg/kg/day during the late phase. These doses are minimal compared to those used for therapy of reflux in pediatric patients (0.1 to 0.5 mg/kg/day).   In these studies, only 1 of 5 infants studied had detectable blood levels of metoclopramide, hence no accumulation or side effects were observed.
T½= 5-6 hours   Oral= 30-100%   Peak= 1-2 hours
LRC=

METOPROLOL

AAP: Compatible

Trade: Toprol XL, Lopressor
Can/Aus/UK: Apo-Metoprolol, Betaloc, Lopressor, Novo-Metoprol, Betaloc, Minax
Specifics: First line choice of beta-blocker for breastfeeding women. Milk levels are minimal. Side effects in infant are minimal.
T½= 3-7 hours   Oral= 40-50%   Peak= 2.5-3 hours
LRC= L3

NAPROXEN

AAP: Compatible

Trade: Anaprox, Naprosyn, Naproxen, Aleve
Can/Aus/UK: Anaprox, Apo-Naproxen, Naprosyn, Naxen, Inza, Naprosyn,

Proxen SR, Synflex
Specifics: Naproxen is a longer half-life NSAID and as such should not be used for long periods in order to prevent buildup in the infant. Infrequent use is not contraindicated, particularly with older infants.
T½= 12-15 hours   Oral= 74-99%   Peak= 2-4 hours
LRC= L3
          L4 for chronic use

NIFEDIPINE   AAP: Compatible

Trade: Adalat, Procardia
Can/Aus/UK: Adalat, Apo-Nifed, Novo-Nifedin, Nu-Nifed, Nifecard, Nyefax, Nefensar XL
Specifics: Milk levels of this calcium channel blocker are quite low. Its use for treating angina is not preferred.
T½= 1.8-7 hours   Oral= 50%   Peak= 45 min-4 hours
LRC= L2

NORTRIPTYLINE   AAP: Not Reviewed

Trade: Aventyl, Pamelor
Can/Aus/UK: Aventyl, Norventyl, Apo-Nortriptyline, Allegron
Specifics: Milk levels of nortriptyline are low to undetectable. No untoward effects have been reported in several studies.
T½= 16-90 hours   Oral= 51%   Peak= 7-8.5 hours
LRC= L2

PROPRANOLOL   AAP: Compatible

Trade: Inderal
Can/Aus/UK: Detensol, Inderal, Novo-Pranol, Deralin, Cardinol
Specifics: Propranolol is an ideal beta-blocker for breastfeeding women. Numerous studies show minimal milk levels and minimal to no side effects in the infant.
T½= 3-5 hours   Oral= 30%   Peak= 60-90 min.
LRC= L3

SUMATRIPTAN SUCCINATE   AAP: Not Reviewed

Trade: Imitrex
Can/Aus/UK: Imitrex, Imigran
Specifics: Two hours following a 6 mg SC dose, milk levels averaged 87.2 µg/L of milk. The oral bioavailability is poor (10-15%), so little is likely absorbed by the infant.
T½= 1.3 hours   Oral= 10-15%   Peak= 12 min.(IM)

204

LRC= L3

VALPROIC ACID

AAP: Compatible

Trade: Depakene, Depakote
Can/Aus/UK: Depakene, Novo-Valproic, Deproic, Epilim, Valpro, Convulex, Epilim
Specifics: Milk levels are low, less than 0.47 mg/Liter of milk.
T½= 14 hours   Oral= Complete   Peak= 1-4 hours
LRC= L2

VERAPAMIL

AAP: Compatible

Trade: Calan, Isoptin, Covera-HS
Can/Aus/UK: Apo-Verap, Isoptin, Novo-Veramil, Anpec, Cordilox, Veracaps SR, Berkatens, Cordilox, Univer
Specifics: Verapamil levels in milk are generally quite low, and side effects have not been noted in breastfeeding infants. Verapamil may also be used in panic and manic attacks. But because it reduces uterine contractility, discontinue prior to delivery.
T½= 3-7 hours   Oral= 90%   Peak= 1-2.2
LRC= L2

Clinical Tips:

Numerous therapies for migraine attacks are available. The choice depends on the severity and frequency of attack, the presence of other conditions (pregnancy, breastfeeding), and patient acceptance. Initial therapy generally starts with oral analgesics, NSAIDs such as ibuprofen or naproxen, or caffeine adjuvant compounds (Fiorinal). Ibuprofen, due to low milk levels, is an ideal NSAID. Naproxen, when used infrequently, is also useful in some patients. Caffeine adjuvant compounds such as butalbital compound (Fiorinal, Fioricet) may work in some patients if used sparingly. Brief use of this barbiturate is unlikely to sedate a breastfeeding infant. More severe headaches may require oral or subcutaneous sumatriptan. Studies show that milk levels of sumatriptan are quite low, and its oral bioavailability is low (10-15%). For long term therapy, propranolol or metoprolol are ideal beta-blockers and have been used in many breastfeeding mothers. Although other beta-blockers have been used (nadolol, atenolol), these have been associated with side effects in infants. Beta-blockers should not be used in patients with low energy levels, depression, congestive heart failure, or asthma. Observe the infant for typical beta-blocker side effects including hypoglycemia, hypotension, weakness, and apnea although these are unlikely. Tricyclic antidepressants (TCAs) have been used for many years. Amitriptyline and nortriptyline are particularly useful for patients with sleep disturbances (insomnia). Side effects of TCAs are common and include dry mouth, constipation, blurred vision, and sedation.

However, their poor penetration into milk make them ideal candidates for chronic pain, including migraine. The anticonvulsant valproic acid is a highly effective treatment for migraines. It is primarily used in a sustained release formulation (divalproex) and plasma levels are maintained as high as 120 μg/mL. It can be safely used in patients with other co-morbid states such as asthma, diabetes, depression, and Raynaud's phenomena conditions that are usually contraindications to the use of beta-blockers. The ergotamine alkaloids (DHE-45, Cafergot, etc) are contraindicated in breastfeeding mothers due to their suppression of prolactin. However, this is not an absolute contraindication, as breastfeeding becomes less dependent on prolactin at 4 to 6 months, and occasional doses later on may not overtly suppress lactation. The limited amount transferred via milk, and the poor oral bioavailability of the ergot alkaloids would limit their clinical effect on an older infant. Recently, the use of intravenous metoclopramide in emergency departments suggests it may be effective alone in treatment of migraine. This use is yet unapproved but would certainly not be contraindicated in breastfeeding mothers.

Suggested Reading:

1.   Diener HC, et al. A practical guide to the management and prevention of migraine. Drugs. 1998 Nov;56(5):811-24. Review.
2.   Ferrari MD. Migraine. Lancet. 1998 Apr 4;351(9108):1043-51. Review.
3.   Young WB, et al. Migraine treatment. Semin Neurol. 1997;17(4):325-33. Review.
4.   Saper JR. Diagnosis and symptomatic treatment of migraine. Headache. 1997;37 Suppl 1:S1-14. Review.
5.   Vinson DR. Treatment patterns of isolated benign headache in US emergency departments. Ann Emerg Med. 2002 Mar;39(3):215-22.

Muscle Spasticity

Principles of Therapy:
Muscle cramps and tetany arise from any number of causes, including sports or occupational muscle injury, hypocalcemia, diabetes mellitus, Parkinson's disease, spinal cord injury, hemodialysis, chemotherapy, and etc. Various drugs have been found to cause cramps and include cimetidine and cholestyramine. Electrolyte deficiencies such as calcium and magnesium are also well known to induce muscle cramping. While correction on the primary etiology is often the wisest course, pharmacotherapy is nevertheless sometimes used along with rest and physical therapy. The medications employed are few, and their mechanism of actions largely unresolved. Because many of these products are poorly efficacious, a risk vs benefit justification is required prior to their use in breastfeeding mothers.

METAXALONE
AAP: Not Reviewed

Trade: Skelaxin
Can/Aus/UK:
Specifics: While we have no breastfeeding data with this product, it produces a low degree of sedation and other major side effects and could possibly be used briefly in breastfeeding mothers.
T½= 2-3 hours   Oral= N/A   Peak= 2 hours
LRC= L3

ORPHENADRINE CITRATE
AAP: Not Reviewed

Trade: Norflex, Banflex, Norgesic, Myotrol
Can/Aus/UK: Disipal, Norflex, Orfenace, Norgesic
Specifics: Orphenadrine is an analog of Benadryl. It is primarily used as a muscle relaxant although its primary effects are anticholinergic. No data are available on its secretion into breastmilk.
T½= 14 hours   Oral= 95%   Peak= 2-4 hours
LRC= L3

QUININE
AAP: Compatible

Trade: Quinamm
Can/Aus/UK:
Specifics: We have two good studies presently that show even after high doses, the amount of quinine in breastmilk is subclinical, less than 1-3 mg daily. Do not use concomitantly with Digoxin.
T½= 11 hours   Oral= 76%   Peak= 1-3 hours
LRC= L2

Clinical Tips:

Quinine is most effective for frequent nocturnal leg cramps. We have two studies that show quinine is quite safe for a breastfeeding mother as the milk levels are quite low. The newer product metaxalone is moderately effective and produces minimal or only occasional sedation. While we have no breastfeeding data on metaxalone, it or quinine are probably preferred. For the most part, these medications have not shown themselves to be much more effective than placebo and rest. Therefore, their use in breastfeeding mothers may not be justified.

Suggested Reading:

1. Chambers HG. The surgical treatment of spasticity. Muscle Nerve Suppl. 1997;6:S121-8. Review.
2. Moore DP. Helping your patients with spasticity reach maximal function. Postgrad Med. 1998 Aug;104(2):123-6, 129-31, 135. Review.
3. Hesse S, et al. Management of spasticity. Curr Opin Neurol. 1997 Dec;10(6):498-501. Review.

Nipple Dermatitis

Principles of Therapy:

The painful nipple is one of the most common complaints of breastfeeding mothers early on and is a major reason for premature weaning. Most nipple irritation is initiated with improper latching of the infant to the nipple. Correction of improper latch and positioning will frequently reduce the pain. The assistance of an experienced lactation consultant to the management of latch difficulties can not be underestimated. Discomfort generally ensues between 3 to 5 days postpartum, followed by steady improvement in most cases. However, in some cases, the pain increases and becomes chronic. While the initial problem may be associated with improper latch, ultimately skin breakdown occurs, and is often associated with superinfections with Candida albicans, Staphylococcus aureus, or both. Initial treatment should be aimed toward providing for a better latch. If the latch is considered adequate, certain medications may be helpful. Skin protectants, such as highly purified lanolin ointments have been used with significant success to prevent skin breakdown in some patients. In some instances, antimicrobials and topical corticosteroids are quite effective and can be used safely in breastfeeding mothers, particularly those with inflamed or infected lesions. Care should be used to limit exposure of the infant to large amounts of topical steroids, particularly high potency steroids.

CLOTRIMAZOLE   AAP: Not Reviewed

Trade: Gyne-Lotrimin, Mycelex, Lotrimin, Femcare
Can/Aus/UK: Canesten, Clotrimaderm, Myclo, Clonea, Hiderm
Specifics: Used for therapy of candida infections, systemic absorption following intravaginal use in minimal (< 3-10%). When placed on the nipple observe for irritation. Use only minimal amounts to avoid systemic absorption in the infant.
T1/2= 3.5-5 hours   Oral= Poor   Peak= 3 hours (oral)
LRC= L1

FLUCONAZOLE   AAP: Not Reviewed

Trade: Diflucan
Can/Aus/UK: Diflucan
Specifics: Published milk levels are quite low and are not sufficient to treat the breastfed infant. Peak levels of fluconazole are 2.93 mg/Liter of milk, or less than 5% of the recommended pediatric dose. The infant will require separate therapy with oral fluconazole or nystatin.
T1/2= 30 hours   Oral= >90%   Peak= 1-2 hours
LRC= L2

GENTIAN VIOLET
AAP: Not Reviewed
Trade: Crystal Violet, Methylrosaniline Chloride, Gentian Violet
Can/Aus/UK:
Specifics: Gentian violet kills candida on contact and is becoming more popular for oral thrush due to resistance to nystatin. Paint infants mouth (including mother's nipple and areola) once daily for no more than 3-7 days with weak (0.5-1%) solutions.
T1/2= N/A   Oral= N/A   Peak= N/A
LRC= L3

MICONAZOLE
AAP: Not Reviewed
Trade: Monistat-Derm, Monistat Vaginal Cream 2%
Can/Aus/UK: Micatin, Monistat, Daktarin, Daktozin, Fungo
Specifics: Good azole topical antifungal. This is an ideal topical choice for the nipple as the oral bioavailability is minimal (< 25%).
T1/2= 20-25 hours   Oral= 25-30%   Peak= Immediate(IV)
LRC=L2

MUPIROCIN OINTMENT
AAP: Not Reviewed
Trade: Bactroban
Can/Aus/UK:
Specifics: Topical antibacterial effective for staphloccal and streptococcal infections. No absorption from topical application.
T1/2= 17-36 min.   Oral= Complete   Peak= N/A
LRC= L1

TRIAMCINOLONE ACETONIDE
AAP: Not Reviewed
Trade: Kenalog, Aristocort, Flutex
Can/Aus/UK: Aristocort, Kenalog, Triaderm, Kenalone
Specifics: Triamcinolone is considered a moderately potent steroid. It is unlikely that systemic absorption by a breastfeeding infant would be significant. Limit amount applied to a minimum.
T1/2= 88 minutes   Oral= Complete   Peak= N/A
LRC= L3

HYDROCORTISONE TOPICAL
AAP: Not Reviewed
Trade: Westcort
Can/Aus/UK: Cortate, Cortone, Aquacort, Dermaid, Egocort, Hycor, Cortef, Dermacort
Specifics: Topical hydrocortisone is a weak corticosteroid and may require several days to work. Absorption in the infant is minimal but use only

minimal amounts.
T1/2= 1-2 hours   Oral= 96%   Peak= N/A
LRC= L2

MOMETASONE   **AAP**: Not Reviewed
  Trade: Elocon Ointment
  Can/Aus/UK:
  Specifics: Topical mometasone is a medium potency steroid. Transfer to
milk is unreported and probably minimal. Mometasone is considered a
moderate potency topical steroid.
  T1/2= N/A   Oral= N/A   Peak= N/A
  LRC= L3

Clinical Tips:

Initial therapy for the sore nipple is to closely evaluate the positioning and latch of the infant. Clinically the inflamed nipple is either due to trauma, inflammation, infection, or all of the above and it may be difficult to discern the offending agent. Simple correction of the latch will provide comfort for the majority of patients. If the infant has thrush, it is likely that the mother's nipple inflammation may be due to infection with *C. Albicans.* In such cases, topical therapy four to five times daily with miconazole (Monistat vaginal), or clotrimazole (Lotrimin) may be useful. (See section on Candida) Some clinicians suggest that clotrimazole may be a topical irritant. In addition, clotrimazole may induce elevated liver enzymes in infants, and oral absorption from the nipple should be minimized. At present, due to major resistance, nystatin is poorly efficacious. In some patients with severe pain radiating into the axilla, oral anti-candida therapy (fluconazole 100-200 mg daily X 14-21 days) in the mother may work effectively. While it has not been documented that candida can infect the ductal tissue of the breast, many of these patients obtain major relief of symptoms with oral antifungal therapy. For the nipple with severe trauma or cracking, topical anti-staphylococcal preparations such as mupirocin (Bactroban) are ideal. Bactroban has limited oral bioavailability. Another anti-infective agent growing in popularity is gentian violet. Topical application of 0.5-1% strength aqueous solutions once daily for 3-7 days is effective in treating superficial candida and bacterial infections of the nipple. It can also be used to paint the fungal lesions in the infant's mouth. Caution, do not overuse gentian violet, as it can damage the mucous membranes if used excessively. Only use weak solutions such as 0.5% to 1% solutions. Patients with severe inflammation often respond to the topical application of moderate strength corticosteroids in combination with mupirocin (Bactroban). Hydrocortisone, triamcinolone or mometasone ointments are ideal. The clinician should warn the mother to limit the amount to an absolute minimum, use them only after the infant has breastfed, and to use them no more than 4-6 times daily. Hydrocortisone ointments, while inexpensive, are only moderately efficacious and slow in acting. Higher potency topical steroids should be avoided. If steroids are overused on the nipple, an infant may show signs of a "steroid" acne around the mouth. Finally, all of these treatments should be considered acute only, chronic use should be strictly avoided. For application to the nipple, ointments are always preferred. While the infant will ingest minor amounts of medication from the nipple, on an acute basis this is seldom enough to produce clinical effects in the infant.

Suggested Reading:

1.   Ward KA, et al. Dermatologic diseases of the breast in young women. Clin Dermatol. 1997 Jan-Feb;15(1):45-52. Review.
2.   Bedinghaus JM. Care of the breast and support of breast-feeding. Prim Care. 1997 Mar;24(1):147-60. Review.

Nipple Vasospasm

Principles of Therapy:

Nipple vasospasm is believed to be a variant of Raynaud's Syndrome in which intense vasospasm of the vessels contiguous with the nipple undergo blanching and cause extreme pain. Classically there is a triphasic color change of the nipple similar to digital ischemia in typical Raynaud's Syndrome. Initially there is a pallor induced by exaggerated sympathetic adrenergic activity, followed by cyanosis and ischemia. Finally rubor, associated with a reflex vasodilation is probably due to release of local cytokines. Symptoms aside from color change include numbness, burning, tingling, and extreme pain. Treatment is largely palliative and is directed toward reducing the conditions that predispose to the symptoms, namely, reducing cold exposure or emotional situations. Preventive measures include warm clothing and avoidance of the following: tobacco in all forms, ergot alkaloids (ergotamine, bromocriptine), beta-blockers, oral contraceptives, and sympathomimetic medications (stimulants, pseudoephedrine, phenylephrine, phenylpropanolamine, etc). Pharmacotherapy is not always effective and often the side effects of the medications preclude continued therapy, particularly with breastfeeding infants.

CAPTOPRIL
AAP: Compatible

Trade: Capoten
Can/Aus/UK: Capoten, Apo-Capto, Novo-Captopril, Acenorm, Enzace, Acepril
Specifics: Milk levels are very low (4.7 µg/L of milk). No adverse effects in 12 infants studied. Avoid in early neonatal periods, infants may be excessively sensitive.
T1/2= 2.2 hours   Oral= 60-75%   Peak= 1 hr.
LRC= L3 if used after 30 days
          L4 if used early postpartum

METHYLDOPA
AAP: Compatible

Trade: Aldomet
Can/Aus/UK: Aldomet, Apo-Methlydopa, Dopamet, Novo-Medopa, Aldopren, Hydopa, Nudopa
Specifics: Reported milk levels are quite low in over 9 patients studied. One case of gynecomastia has been reported (personal communication).
T1/2= 105 min.   Oral= 25-50%   Peak= 3-6 hours
LRC= L2

NIFEDIPINE   AAP: Compatible
Trade: Adalat, Procardia
Can/Aus/UK: Adalat, Apo-Nifed, Novo-Nifedin, Nu-Nifed, Nifecard, Nyefax, Nefensar XL
Specifics: Milk levels of this calcium channel blocker are quite low. Doses for Raynaud's syndrome vary from 30-60 mg per day in sustained release formulations.
T1/2= 1.8-7 hours   Oral= 50%   Peak= 45 min-4 hours
LRC= L2

TERBUTALINE   AAP: Compatible
Trade: Bricanyl, Brethine
Can/Aus/UK: Bricanyl
Specifics: Following the oral administration in mothers, milk levels were minimal. No untoward effects were noted in breastfed infants.
T1/2= 14 hours   Oral= 33-50%   Peak= 5-30 min.
LRC= L2

Clinical Tips:

Initially, preventive measures such as evaluation of the infant's latch (poor positioning and attachment), and other breastfeeding factors must be explored. Patients should be advised to avoid stressful situations when breastfeeding, and to avoid cold environments. Failing this, pharmacologic therapy is indicated in those individuals for whom preventive measure have been ineffective. While numerous medications are effective, all of the sympatholytics, alpha-adrenergic blockers, beta-receptor agonists, and calcium channel blockers may create intolerable side effects for the patient. At present, most agree that the newer slow-channel calcium channel blockers are greatly preferred due to efficacy and minimal side effects. These act by reducing vasospasm and vasoconstriction by reducing calcium influx into the vascular smooth muscle cell. Of these, nifedipine is greatly preferred because it has the most potent peripheral action and its concentration in human milk is minimal. The recommended starting dose is 10 mg orally three times daily, increasing the dose in a stepwise fashion as dictated by clinical response. Experience with long-acting dosage forms is limited, but they are expected to be equally efficacious. While other agents have been used successfully, they are somewhat more risky in a breastfeeding mother. ACE inhibitors such as captopril has been used but are only about 30% effective in Raynaud's syndrome. In addition, ACE inhibitors should be used cautiously during the perinatal period (first 1-2 months postpartum) due to risk of hypotension in the infant. Older infants are less sensitive to this exaggerated hypotension from ACE inhibitors. Methyldopa is about 50% effective and several studies show low milk levels. Although nicotinic acid is marginally effective (<40%) its use in high doses could be problematic for a breastfed infant (liver damage).   Alpha-adrenergic blockers have not been studied in breastfeeding mothers, but due to their high potency they are probably too toxic to risk (prazosin, phenoxybenzamine). There are numerous other medications that are poorly efficacious and have not been studied in breastfeeding mothers. These include: griseofulvin, papaverine, nitrates, guanethidine, reserpine, prostaglandins (PGI2, PGE1), thyroid, dextran, and pentoxifylline.

Suggested Reading:

1.   Coates M. Nipple Pain Related to Vasospasm in the Nipple? J Hum Lact. 1992; 8(3):153.
2.   Lawlor-Smith LS, Lawlor-Smith CL. Vasopasm of the Nipple - A manifestation of Raynaud's Phenomenon. BMJ 1997;314:644-645.
3.   Rodheffer RJ, Rommer JA, Wigley F, Smith CR. Controlled Double- Blind Trial of Nifedipine in the Treatment of Raynaud's Phenomenon. N Engl J Med. 1983; 308: 880-883.
4.   Corbin DOC, Wood DA, MacIntyre CCA, Housley E. A Randomised Double Blind Cross-Over Trial of Nifedipine in the Treatment of Primary Raynaud's Phenomenon. Eur Heart J 1986; 7;165-170.
5.   Kahan A, Weber S, Amor B, et al Calcium Entry Blocking Agents in Digital Vasospasm (Raynaud's Phenomenon). Eur Heart J. 1983; 4 (Suppl C): 123.
6.   Ehrenkranz RA, Ackerman BA, Hulse JD. Nifedipine Transfer into Human Milk. The Journal of Pediatrics. March 1989; 478-480.

Pain

Principles of Therapy:

Pain is the most common symptom causing patients to seek medical attention. Proper treatment of pain depends largely on the careful diagnosis and source of the pain. As such, the medications used are largely determined by the source and cause of pain. The following medications are those generally used as analgesics for a variety of pain. More complete descriptions of pain by syndrome such as 'Migraine Headaches' are provided under their specific categories.

ACETAMINOPHEN
AAP: Compatible

Trade: Tempra, Tylenol, Paracetamol
Can/Aus/UK: Apo-Acetaminophen, Tempra, Tylenol, Paracetamol, Panadol, Dymadon, Calpol
Specifics: Only minimal amounts are secreted in milk.
T½= 2 hours   Oral= >85%   Peak= 0.5-2 hours
LRC= L1

ASPIRIN
AAP: Give with caution

Trade: Excedrin, Ecotrin
Can/Aus/UK: Ecotrin
Specifics: Aspirin levels in human milk are exceedingly low. Occasional use in breastfeeding mothers is not absolutely contraindicated. It should never be used when the infant is sick or febrile due to its relationship with Reye's syndrome.
T½= 2.5-7 hours   Oral= 80-100%   Peak= 1-2 hours
LRC= L3

CODEINE
AAP: Compatible

Trade: Empirin #3 # 4, Tylenol # 3 # 4
Can/Aus/UK: Paveral, Penntuss, Actacode, Codalgin, Codral, Panadeine, Veganin, Kaodene, Teropin
Specifics: Breastmilk levels of codeine are minimal if the dose is kept less than 60 mg.
T½= 2.9 hours   Oral= Complete   Peak= 0.5-1 hr.
LRC= L3

FLURBIPROFEN   AAP: Not Reviewed

Trade: Ansaid, Froben, Ocufen
Can/Aus/UK: Ansaid, Froben, Ocufen
Specifics: Reported milk levels in two studies are reported to be exceedingly low.
T½= 3.8-5.7 hours   Oral= Complete   Peak= 1.5 hours
LRC= L2

HYDROCODONE   AAP: Not Reviewed

Trade: Lortab, Vicodin
Can/Aus/UK:
Specifics: Although we have minimal data on hydrocodone's transfer to milk, its use in breastfeeding women is widespread and only occasional sedation has been reported.
T½= 3.8 hours   Oral= Complete   Peak= 1.3 hours
LRC= L3

IBUPROFEN   AAP: Compatible

Trade: Advil, Nuprin, Motrin, Pediaprofen
Can/Aus/UK: Actiprofen, Advil, Amersol, Motrin, ACT-3, Brufen, Nurofen, Rafen
Specifics: Ibuprofen is an ideal NSAID for breastfeeding mother due to short half-life and minimal breastmilk levels.
T½= 1.8-2.5 hours   Oral= 80%   Peak= 1-2 hours
LRC= L1

KETOROLAC   AAP: Compatible

Trade: Toradol, Acular
Can/Aus/UK: Acular, Toradol
Specifics: In a study of 10 patients receiving 10 mg PO four times daily, ketorolac was undetectable in 4 milk samples and exceedingly low in the other 6 patient samples (5.2-7.3 µg/L). While the manufacturer does not approve the use of ketorolac in breastfeeding mothers, the levels in breastmilk are incredibly low, far too low to induce clinical effects in a breastfeeding infant. No evidence of untoward effects in infants has been published.
T½= 2.4-8.6 hours   Oral= >81%   Peak= 0.5 - 1 hr.
LRC= L2

MEPERIDINE

AAP: Not Reviewed

Trade: Demerol
Can/Aus/UK:
Specifics: Meperidine (pethidine) has a long half-life active metabolite, that when used prenatally can cause prolonged sedation in the neonate. Infrequent or acute use of meperidine such as in a dental procedure is not contraindicated.

T½= 3.2 hours   Oral= <50%   Peak=30-50 min.(IM)
LRC= L2
          L3 if used early postpartum

MORPHINE

AAP: Compatible

Trade: Morphine
Can/Aus/UK: Epimorph, Morphitec, M.O.S. MS Contin, Statex, Morphalgin, Ordine, Anamorph, Kapanol, Oramorph, Sevredol
Specifics: Transfer of morphine to milk has been reported to be minimal, with exception of one report. Numerous other reports suggest transfer to milk is low and use in the perinatal period is believed safe. Clinical studies suggest morphine, due to its first-pass pickup by the liver, to be an ideal analgesic for breastfeeding mothers.

T½= 1.5-2 hours   Oral= 26%   Peak= 0.5-1 hours
LRC= L3

NAPROXEN

AAP: Compatible

Trade: Anaprox, Naprosyn, Naproxen, Aleve
Can/Aus/UK: Anaprox, Apo-Naproxen, Naprosyn, Naxen, Inza, Proxen SR, Synflex
Specifics: Naproxen is a longer half-life NSAID and should not be used for long periods. Infrequent or occasional use is not contraindicated particularly with older infants.

T½= 12-15 hours   Oral= 74-99%   Peak= 2-4 hours
LRC= L3
          L4 for chronic use

Clinical Tips:

The control of pain largely depends on the source. For severe pain, the opioids are preferred and include morphine, codeine, hydrocodone, and lastly meperidine. In several studies, morphine seems to be an ideal analgesic for breastfeeding mothers as its bioavailability (via milk) is low and it seems to produce the least sedation in breastfed infants. Meperidine(pethidine) has a long half-life 'active' metabolite and may not be a preferred analgesic pre- or postnatally. Morphine and the codeine derivatives such as hydrocodone have been used extensively in breastfeeding women with only occasional neonatal sedation reported. For rheumatic pain, the NSAID family is ideal. Of this family, ibuprofen is preferred, due to poor transfer into milk and its safety in infants. Longer half-life NSAIDS such as naproxen should only be used for short periods, thus eliminating accumulation in the infant's plasma. Ketorolac (Toradol) is somewhat controversial as the manufacturer's information suggests it should not be used in breastfeeding women. However, an excellent study clearly shows that milk levels are far subclinical, and ketorolac should be an ideal NSAID for use in certain breastfeeding women. The transfer of flurbiprofen into milk is reported to be very low and could be used cautiously.

Suggested Reading:

1. Boynton CS, Dick CF, Mayor GH. NSAIDs: an overview. J.Clin. Pharmacol. 1988; 28:512-517.
2. Beaver WT. Combination Analgesics. Am. J. Med. 1984; 77:38-53.
3. The International Association for the Study of Pain, Subcommittee on Taxonomy. Classification of chronic pain: descriptions of chronic pain syndromes and definitions of pain terms. Pain 1986; 3(suppl): S1-S226.
4. Wischnik A, Manth SM, Lloyd J. The excretion of ketorolac tromethamine into breast milk after multiple oral dosing. Eur. J. Clin. Pharm. 36:521-524, 1989.

Pelvic Inflammatory Disease

Principles of Therapy:

Pelvic Inflammatory Disease (PID) is used to describe a spectrum of inflammatory diseases of the upper female genital tract including non-puerperal endometritis, peritonitis, salpingitis, and tubo-ovarian abscess. Sexually transmitted organisms such as *Neisseria gonorrhoeae* and *Chlamydia trachomatis*, may instigate the infection though once established this is a polymicrobial infection often involving organisms from vaginal flora. *Escherichia coli* and bacteroides are other commonly involved organisms. Clinical diagnosis of PID is imperfect. Laparoscopy can provide a more accurate diagnosis but remains an invasive surgical procedure that is usually reserved for cases unresponsive to antibiotic therapy or with unclear diagnosis. Risk factors for development of PID include: multiple sexual partners, a new partner, unprotected intercourse, and a history of an untreated sexually transmitted disease. Diagnostic criteria are imperfect. Minimal criteria for diagnosis include lower abdominal pain, adenexal tenderness, and cervical motion tenderness with no other apparent cause for these symptoms. Additional criteria to support this diagnosis include fever, abnormal vaginal discharge, and documentation of cervical infection with chlamydia or gonorrhea. Pelvic ultrasound may also be useful in cases of suspected tubo-ovarian abscess. Any treatment scheme must cover chlamydia and gonorrhea though other organisms are frequently involved including various gram positive and gram negative species. The diagnosis of PID is even more challenging as many cases of PID have few or no symptoms. The classic clinical symptoms of acute PID including lower abdominal pain, fever, adnexal tenderness or mass, purulent discharge from the cervix, elevated white cell count, and sedimentation rate is rarely found. Treatment of PID is largely based on the use of multiple antibiotics regimens to ensure broad spectrum coverage. Therapy can be given either in an inpatient or outpatient setting. Criteria for hospitalization include inability to tolerate oral medications due to nausea and vomiting, uncertain diagnosis, evidence of peritonitis or pelvic abscess, suspected non-compliance, immunodeficiency, and failed outpatient therapy. PID has many late sequelae including infertility, ectopic pregnancy and chronic pelvic pain.

AMPICILLIN / SULBACTAM   AAP: Not Reviewed
Trade: Unasyn,
Can/Aus/UK: Magnapen
Specifics: Ampicillin+sulbactam is an antibiotic combination composed of ampicillin, and sulbactam, a beta-lactamase inhibitor. The addition of sulbactam extends the antimicrobial spectrum of ampicillin. Ampicillin levels in milk are generally less than 1 mg/Liter.

T½= 1.3 hours   Oral= 50%   Peak= 1-2 hours
LRC= L1

AZITHROMYCIN

AAP: Not Reviewed

Trade: Zithromax
Can/Aus/UK: Zithromax
Specifics: Azithromycin levels in milk are very low. In one study of a patient who received 1 gm initially, followed by two 500mg doses at 24 hr intervals, the concentration of azithromycin in breastmilk varied from 0.64 mg/L (initially) to 2.8 mg/L on day 3.

T1/2= 48-68 hours   Oral= 37%   Peak= 3-4 hours
LRC= L2

CEFTRIAXONE

AAP: Not Reviewed

Trade: Rocephin
Can/Aus/UK: Rocephin
Specifics: Small amounts are transferred into milk (3-4% of maternal serum level). Following a 1 gm IM dose, breastmilk levels were approximately 0.5-0.7 mg/L between 4-8 hours. The estimated mean milk levels at steady state were 3-4 mg/L. Another source indicates that following a 2 gm/d dose and at steady state, approximately 4.4 % of dose penetrates into milk. In this study, the maximum breastmilk concentration was 7.89 mg/L after prolonged therapy (7days). Using this data, the weight-adjusted relative infant dose would only be 0.35% of the maternal dose. Poor oral absorption of ceftriaxone would further limit systemic absorption by the infant.

T½= 7.3 hours   Oral= Poor   Peak= 1 hour
LRC= L2

CEFOXITIN

AAP: Compatible

Trade: Mefoxin
Can/Aus/UK: Mefoxin
Specifics: Milk levels are very low, and oral bioavailability is poor. In a study of 2-3 women who received 1000 mg I.V., only trace amounts were reported in milk over 6 hours. In a group of 5 women who received an IM injection of 2000 mg, milk levels the highest milk levels were reported at 4 hours after dose. The maternal plasma levels varied from 22.5 at 2 hours to 77.6 µg/mL at 4 hours. Maternal milk levels ranged from < 0.25 to 0.65 mg/L.

T1/2= 0.7-1.1 hours   Oral= Poor   Peak= 20-30 min (IM)
LRC= L1

CIPROFLOXACIN

AAP: Approved

Trade: Cipro, Ciloxan
Can/Aus/UK: Cipro, Ciloxan, Ciproxin
Specifics: In one study of 10 women who received 750 mg every 12 hours, milk levels of ciprofloxacin ranged from 3.79 mg/L at 2 hours post-dose to 0.02 mg/L at 24 hours. In another study of a single patient receiving one 500

mg tablet daily at bedtime, the concentrations in maternal serum and breastmilk were 0.21 µg/mL, and 0.98 µg/mL, respectively. Plasma levels were undetectable (< 0. 03 µg/mL) in the infant. The dose to the 4 month-old infant was estimated to be 0.92 mg/day or 0.15 mg/kg/day. No adverse effects were noted in this infant. There has been one reported case of severe pseudomembranous colitis in an infant of one mother who self-medicated with ciprofloxacin for 6 days.

T½= 4.1 hours   Oral= 50-85%   Peak= 0.5-2.3 hours
LRC= L4

CLINDAMYCIN   AAP: Compatible
Trade: Cleocin
Can/Aus/UK: Dalacin, Clindatech, Cleocin
Specifics: Following oral doses of 300 mg every 6 hours, the breastmilk levels averaged 1.0 to 1.7 mg/L at 1.5 to 7 hours after dosing. One case of pseudomembranous colitis has been reported following high-dose IV therapy.

T1/2= 2.9 hours   Oral= 90%   Peak=45-60 min (oral)
LRC= L3

DOXYCYCLINE   AAP: Not Reviewed
Trade: Doxychel, Vibramycin
Can/Aus/UK: Apo-Doxy, Doxycin, Vibramycin, Vibra-Tabs, Doryx, Doxylin, Doxylar
Specifics: Milk levels are low (< 0.77 mg/L). Oral bioavailability is reduced (20%) in milk but not eliminated. Limited use is unlikely to produce side effects.

T1/2= 15-25 hours   Oral= 90-100%   Peak= 1.5-4 hours
LRC= L3
          L4 if used chronically

GENTAMYCIN   AAP: Not Reviewed
Trade: Garamycin
Can/Aus/UK: Alocomicin, Cidomycin, Garamycin, Garatec,Palacos, Septopal
Specifics: The oral absorption of gentamicin (<1%) is generally nil with exception of premature neonates where small amounts may be absorbed.1 In one study of 10 women given 80 mg three times daily IM for 5 days postpartum, milk levels were measured on day 4. Gentamicin levels in milk were 0.42, 0.48, 0.49, and 0.41 mg/L at 1, 3, 5, and 7 hours respectively. The milk/plasma ratios were 0.11 at one hour and 0.44 at 7 hours. Plasma gentamicin levels in neonates were small, were found in only 5 of the 10 neonates, and averaged 0.41 µg/ml. The authors estimate that daily ingestion via breastmilk would be 307 µg for a 3.6 kg neonate (normal neonatal dose =

2.5 mg/kg every 12 hours).
T1/2= 2-3 hours   Oral= < 1%   Peak= Immediate
LRC= L2

METRONIDAZOLE   **AAP**: May be of concern
Trade: Flagyl, Metizol, Trikacide, Protostat
Can/Aus/UK: Apo-Metronidazole, Flagyl, NeoMetric, Novo-Nidazol,
Metrozine, Rozex
Specifics: Milk levels are low. Maximum reported levels are 15 μg/mL of
milk. Infant's plasma levels are approximately 10% of maternal levels. No
untoward effects have been reported in numerous studies.
T1/2= 8.5 hours   Oral= Complete   Peak= 2-4 hours
LCR= L2

OFLOXACIN   **AAP**: Not Reviewed
Trade: Floxin
Can/Aus/UK: Floxin, Ocuflox, Tarivid
Specifics: In one study in lactating women who received 400 mg oral doses
twice daily, drug concentrations in breastmilk averaged 0.05-2.41 mg/L in
milk (24 hours and 2 hours post-dose respectively). Milk levels are much
lower than ciprofloxacin levels.
T1/2= 5-7 hours   Oral= 98 %   Peak= 0.5-2 hours
LCR= L3

Clinical Tips:

Treatment regimens vary enormously depending on the suitability of oral verses
intravenous therapy. Typical intravenous therapy involves cefotetan or cefoxitin
combined with doxycycline. Alternatively clindamycin and gentamycin can be used.
There is no advantage to intravenous doxycycline if oral medication can be tolerated
and infusion is associated with significant pain. Cefoxitin 2 gm every 6 hours or
cefotetan 2 gm IV every 12 hours plus doxycycline 100 mg IV/PO every 12 hours is
suitable. Many alternative intravenous treatment regimens are acceptable involving
the use of ofloxacin, metronidazole, ampicillin with sulbactam and ciprofloxacin.
The primary oral regimen is ofloxacin 400 mg orally twice daily for 14 days plus
metronidazole 500 mg orally twice daily for 14 days. While fluoroquinolones are
not ideal candidates for breastfeeding mothers, ofloxacin milk levels are documented
to be low. Another oral regimen is ceftriaxone 250 mg IM plus doxycycline 100 mg
twice daily for 14 days. Azithromycin can be substituted for doxycycline regimens
in hypersensitive individuals.

Suggested Reading:

1.   Gilbert DN, Moellering RC, Sande MA. The Sandford guide to antimicrobial therapy
      1998.

2. Jacobson L, Westrom L. Objectivized diagnosis of pelvic inflammatory disease: Diagnostic and prognostic value of routine laparoscopy. Am. J. Obstet. Gynecol. 1969; 105:1088-1098.
3. Ledger WJ. Anaerobic infections. Am. J. Obstet. Gynecol 1975; 123:111-118.

Peptic Ulcer Disease

Principles of Therapy:
The normal gastric and duodenal mucosa are remarkably capable of defending against injury from the acid of peptic activity in gastric fluids. It is now clear that the two most important insults predisposing to peptic ulceration (PUD) are infection with *Helicobacter pylori* (HP) and the use of nonsteroidal anti-inflammatory drugs (NSAIDS). Although other forms of ulceration exist such as with Crohn's disease, extreme acid hypersecretion, etc, these are rare. The medications used for PUD consist of acid suppressors such as the H_2 blockers (famotidine, ranitidine, etc.) or the proton-pump inhibitors (omeprazole, lansoprazole), coating agents (e.g. sucralfate), antacids, and antibiotics for treating HP infections.

AMOXICILLIN
AAP: Compatible

Trade: Larotid, Amoxil
Can/Aus/UK: Amoxil, Apo-Amoxi, Novamoxin, Alphamox, Moxacin, Cilamox, Betamox
Specifics: Amoxicillin levels in milk are low and average 0.9 mg/Liter of milk or lower.
T½= 1.7 hours   Oral= 89%   Peak= 1.5 hours
LRC= L1

BISMUTH SUBSALICYLATE
AAP: May be of concern

Trade: Pepto-Bismol
Can/Aus/UK:
Specifics: Bismuth salts are poorly absorbed from the maternal GI tract. Significant transfer into milk is highly unlikely.
T½= N/A   Oral= Poor   Peak= N/A
LRC= L3

CLARITHROMYCIN
AAP: Not Reviewed

Trade: Biaxin
Can/Aus/UK: Biaxin, Klacid
Specifics: Levels in milk are unknown, but most macrolide antibiotics are cleared for use in breastfeeding mothers.
T½= 5-7 hours   Oral= 50%   Peak= 1.7 hours
LRC= L2

FAMOTIDINE
AAP: Not Reviewed

Trade: Pepcid, Axid-AR, Pepcid-AC
Can/Aus/UK: Pepcid, Apo-Famotidine, Novo-Famotidine, Amfamox, Pepcidine
Specifics: Reported milk levels are very low (72µg/L).
T½= 2.5-3.5 hours   Oral= 50%   Peak= 1-3.5 hours
LRC= L2

ESOMEPRAZOLE
AAP: Not Reviewed

Trade: Nexium
Can/Aus/UK: Nexium
Specifics: Esomeprazole is the L isomer of omeprazole (Prilosec). See omeprazole below.
T½= 1 hr.   Oral= 30-40%   Peak= 0.5-3.5 hours
LRC= L2

LANSOPRAZOLE
AAP: Not Reviewed

Trade: Prevacid, Prevpac
Can/Aus/UK: Prevacid, Prevpac
Specifics: Structurally similar to omeprazole, it is very unstable in stomach acid and to a large degree is denatured by acidity of the infant's stomach. A new study shows milk levels of omeprazole are minimal (see omeprazole) and it is likely milk levels of lansoprazole are small as well. Although there are no studies of lansoprazole in breastfeeding mothers, transfer to milk and its oral absorption (via milk) is likely to be minimal in a breastfed infant. Prevpac contains Lansoprazole, Amoxicillin, and Clarithromycin. It is primarily indicated for treatment of *H.Pylori* infections which cause stomach ulcers.
T½= hours   Oral= Nil(in infant)   Peak= 1.7 hours
LRC= L3

METRONIDAZOLE
AAP: May be of concern

Trade: Flagyl, Metizol, Trikacide, Protostat
Can/Aus/UK: Apo-Metronidazole, Flagyl, NeoMetric, Novo-Nidazol, Metrozine, Rozex
Specifics: Milk levels are low. Maximum reported levels are 15 µg/mL of milk. Infant's plasma levels are approximately 10% of maternal levels. No untoward effects have been reported in numerous studies.
T½= 8.5 hours   Oral= Complete   Peak= 2-4 hours
LRC= L2

NIZATIDINE

AAP: Not Reviewed

Trade: Axid
Can/Aus/UK: Axid, Apo-Nizatidine, Tazac
Specifics: Only minimal amounts are transferred to milk (< 0.1% of maternal dose).
T½= 1.5 hours   Oral= 94%   Peak= 0.5-3 hours
LRC= L2

OMEPRAZOLE

AAP: Not Reviewed

Trade: Prilosec
Can/Aus/UK: Prilosec, Losec
Specifics: Omeprazole is a potent inhibitor of gastric acid secretion.   In a study of one patient receiving 20 mg omeprazole daily, the maternal serum concentration was 950 nM at 240 min.   The breastmilk concentration of omeprazole began to rise minimally at 90 minutes after ingestion but peaked after 180 minutes at only 58 nM or less than 7% of the highest serum level. Omeprazole milk levels were essentially flat over 4 hours of observation. Omeprazole is extremely acid labile with a half-life of 10 minutes at pH values below pH 4.   Virtually all omeprazole ingested via milk would probably be destroyed in the stomach of the infant prior to absorption.
T½= 1 hr.   Oral= 30-40%   Peak= 0.5-3.5 hours
LRC= L2

RANITIDINE

AAP: Not Reviewed

Trade: Zantac
Can/Aus/UK: Apo-Ranitidine, Novo-Ranidine, Zantac, Nu-Ranit
Specifics: Following a dose of 150 mg for four doses, concentrations in breastmilk were 0.72, 2.6, and 1.5 mg/L at 1.5, 5.5 and 12 hours respectively. Although the milk/plasma ratios are quite high, using this data an infant consuming 1 L of milk daily would ingest less than 2.6 mg/24 hours. This amount is quite small considering the pediatric dose currently recommended is 2-4 mg/kg/24 hours.
T½= 2-3 hours   Oral= 50%   Peak= 1-3 hours
LRC= L2

SUCRALFATE

AAP: Not Reviewed

Trade: Carafate
Can/Aus/UK: Sulcrate, Novo-Sucralate, Nu-Sucralfate, Carafate, SCF, Ulcyte, Antepsin
Specifics: Sucralfate acts topically to cover the mucosal lining of the esophagus, stomach, and duodenum.   Less than 5% is absorbed and it is

unlikely to penetrate milk.
T½= N/A   Oral= < 5%   Peak= N/A
LRC= L2

TETRACYCLINE   AAP: Compatible

Trade: Achromycin, Sumycin, Terramycin
Can/Aus/UK: Achromycin, Aureomycin, Tetracyn, Mysteclin, Tetrex, Tetrachel
Specifics: Milk levels are low, and oral bioavailability in milk is low. In a study of 5 lactating women receiving 500 mg PO four times daily, the breastmilk concentrations ranged from 0.43 mg/L to 2.58 mg/L. Levels in infants were below the limit of detection. Chronic use over months may not be advisable due to dental staining.
T½= 6-12 hours   Oral= 75%   Peak= 1.5-4 hours
LRC= L2

Clinical Tips:
Therapy of gastric ulceration largely depends on etiology. NSAID ulcers should be treated by withdrawal of the offending agent and adding an H2 blocker such as famotidine. Peptic ulceration of *H. pylori* etiology requires up to two weeks of therapy with omeprazole and one of numerous antibiotic regimens. Antibiotics in common use include clarithromycin, tetracycline, metronidazole, amoxicillin, and others. Due to the emergence of resistance, monotherapy is not considered a treatment of choice for eradicating H. pylori.   For this reason, the above antibiotics/proton pump inhibitors are used in combination, such as clarithromycin + omeprazole + metronidazole (MOC therapy), or Pepto-Bismol + metronidazole+ tetracycline or amoxicillin.   Recently, shorter course BID therapy (7 days) with omeprazole, metronidazole or amoxicillin, and clarithromycin has shown promising results (90% eradication). Although most of the above antibiotics transfer poorly into human milk, some changes in the infant's GI flora may result in diarrhea (rarely).

Currently, eight H. pylori treatment regimens are approved by the Food and Drug Administration (FDA).   These are not necessarily approved by the FDA for breastfeeding women but all are suitable.

Treatment Protocols for H. Pylori

1. Omeprazole 40 mg QD + clarithromycin 500 mg TID x 2 weeks, then omeprazole 20 mg QD x 2 weeks
2. Ranitidine bismuth citrate (RBC) 400 mg BID + clarithromycin 500 mg TID x 2 weeks, then RBC 400 mg BID x 2 weeks
3. Bismuth subsalicylate (Pepto Bismol®) 525 mg QID + metronidazole 250 mg QID + tetracycline 500 mg QID* x 2 weeks + H2 receptor antagonist therapy as directed x 4 weeks
4. Lansoprazole 30 mg BID + amoxicillin 1 g BID + clarithromycin 500 mg TID x 10 days
5. Lansoprazole 30 mg TID + amoxicillin 1 g TID x 2 weeks**
6. Rantidine bismuth citrate 400 mg BID + clarithromycin 500 mg BID x 2 weeks, then RBC 400 mg BID x 2 weeks
7. Omeprazole 20 mg BID + clarithromycin 500 mg BID + amoxicillin 1 g BID x 10 days
8. Lansoprazole 30 mg BID + clarithromycin 500 mg BID + amoxicillin 1 g BID x 10 days

*Although not FDA approved, amoxicillin has been substituted for tetracycline for patients for whom tetracycline is not recommended.

**This dual therapy regimen has restrictive labeling. It is indicated for patients who are either allergic or intolerant to clarithromycin or for infections with known or suspected resistance to clarithromycin.

Suggested Reading:

1. Hunt RH. Peptic ulcer disease: defining the treatment strategies in the era of Helicobacter pylori. Am J Gastroenterol. 1997 Apr;92(4 Suppl):36S-40S; discussion 40S-43S. Review.
2. Sarner A, et al. Peptic ulcer disease: paradigms lost. Mt Sinai J Med. 1996 Oct-Nov;63(5-6):387-98. Review.
3. Taniguchi DK, et al. Helicobacter pylori and peptic ulcer disease: issues for primary care providers. Compr Ther. 1996 Jul;22(7):434-9. Review.
4. CDC website: http://www.cdc.gov/ulcer/md.htm#treatment

Psoriasis

Principles of Therapy:
Psoriasis is a chronic, recurrent hereditary disease characterized by well-circumscribed, dry, scaling papules and plaques. It varies in severity from 1 or 2 lesions to widespread scaling papules with acute arthritis. Onset is gradual. Factors precipitating psoriasis attacks include stress, local trauma, severe sunburn, irritation, drugs such as chloroquine, lithium, beta-blockers and withdrawal from systemic corticosteroid therapy. Psoriasis most often occurs on the scalp, elbows and knees, back and buttocks. The lesions are sharply demarcated, usually non-pruritic, over-covered with shiny, opalescent scaling. Treatment involves three common modalities: topical treatment, ultraviolet radiation, and rarely systemic medications.

FLUTICASONE TOPICAL   AAP: Not Reviewed

Trade: Cutivate
Can/Aus/UK:
Specifics: Fluticasone is a medium-potency topical corticosteroid. However topical fluticasone is poorly absorbed transcutaneously, and even less absorbed orally (<1%). Although expensive, it would be an ideal product for use in breastfeeding mothers, especially for large area use.
T½=   7.8 hours   Oral= <1 %   Peak=
LRC= L3

TRIAMCINOLONE ACETONIDE   AAP: Not Reviewed

Trade: Flutex, Kenalog, Aristocort
Can/Aus/UK: Aristocort, Kenalog, Triaderm, Kenalone, Adcortyl
Specifics: Triamcinolone is considered a moderately potent steroid. Percutaneous absorption is minimal. It is unlikely that systemic absorption by a breastfeeding infant would be significant. Limit amount applied to a minimum.
T½= 88 minutes   Oral= Complete   Peak= N/A
LRC= L3

HYDROCORTISONE TOPICAL   AAP: Not Reviewed

Trade: Westcort
Can/Aus/UK: Cortate, Cortone, Emo-Cort, Aquacort, Dermaid, Egocort, Hycor, Cortef, Dermacort
Specifics: Topical hydrocortisone is relatively impotent and is seldom used in psoriasis. Most topical steroids are no longer recommended for psoriasis.

T½= 1-2 hours   Oral= 96%   Peak= N/A
LRC= L2

ANTHRALIN   AAP: Not Reviewed

Trade: Anthra-Derm, Drithocreme, Dritho-Scalp, Micanol
Can/Aus/UK:
Specifics: Systemic absorption following topical use is minimal. Use on large surface areas, or on areola or nipple, may require brief interruption.
T½= Brief   Oral= Complete   Peak= N/A
LRC= L3

TACROLIMUS TOPICAL   AAP: Not Reviewed

Trade: Prograf, Protopic
Can/Aus/UK: Protopic
Specifics: Tacrolimus is an immunosuppressant formerly known as SK506. In one report of 21 mothers who received tacroliumus while pregnant, milk concentrations in colostrum averaged 0.79 ng/mL and varied from 0.3 to 1.9 nanograms/mL.   Using this data and an average daily milk intake of 150 mL/kg, the average dose to the infant per day via milk would be < 0.1 µg/kg/day. Because the oral bioavailability is poor (<32%), an infant would likely ingest less than 100 ng/kg/day.   Recently the FDA has approved a topical form of tacrolimus (Protopic) for use in moderate to severe eczema, in those for whom standard eczema therapies are deemed inadvisable. Absorption via skin is minimal. In a study of 46 adult patients af multiple doses, plasma levels ranged from undetectable to 20 ng/mL, with 45 of the patients have peak blood concentrations less than 5 ng/mL. In another study, the peak blood levels averaged 1.6 ng/mL which is significantly less than the therapeutic range in kidney transplantation(7-20 ng/mL). While the absolute transcutaneous bioavailability is unknown it is apparently very low. Combined with the poor oral bioavailability of this product it is not likely a breastfed infant will receive enough following topical use
T½= 34.2 hours   Oral= 14-32%   Peak=1.6 hours
LRC= L3

TAZAROTENE   AAP: Not Reviewed

Trade: Tazorac
Can/Aus/UK:
Specifics: Transcutaneous absorption of tazarotene is low (<1 %). Because it is metabolized to a retinoid, it could penetrate milk but the concentrations would likely be subclinical. Virtually none is detectable in the plasma compartment of the user.

T½= 18 hours   Oral= N/A   Peak= N/A
LRC= L3

Clinical Tips:

Therapy of psoriasis normally starts with the use of topical steroids although it may be inadvisable. Two factors are of major concern in the choice of treatment: one is the severity of the lesions and secondly, the surface area of the body affected. Topical steroids rarely return the skin to a normal state and when discontinued the psoriatic lesion rapidly recurs. Further, after continued treatment, a steroid-resistant state ensues with permanent atrophy of the skin and a more aggressive psoriatic lesion. Treatment of large surface areas with steroids can induce adrenal suppression. General consensus is that systemic steroids have no place in the treatment of psoriasis, because rebound spreading of the disease is a major result. However, steroids can be used initially if 'pulse therapy' is employed. Basically high potency steroids are used but only on two days of the week such as Saturday and Sunday. This prevents the rapid tachyphylaxis to steroids and can help many patients. Newer therapies (newer formulations) using anthralin have increased in popularity because it can clear psoriasis and produce remissions for many months without continued treatment. Anthralin is poorly absorbed through the skin. Studies show plasma levels are brief and hardly detectable. Milk levels of anthralin have not been determined, but are probably very low. Tar is an effective treatment, but it is messy to use, and it may be carcinogenic in humans over time. Unfortunately, the safer, refined tar preparations are poorly effective. Phototherapy with lubrication is an effective treatment of psoriasis. Almost 95% of patients will benefit from ultraviolet B irradiation when applied under medical supervision in correct doses. Lubrication is applied to each lesion prior to irradiation as it facilitates penetration. Systemic therapy with methotrexate is highly effective but has two major problems. One is that it is highly teratogenic, it suppresses bone marrow, and may be sequestered in the GI cells of infants for long periods. And two, it appears to alter the nature of psoriasis, ultimately making it a more severe and aggressive disease with each rebound. Hence the type and severity of the disease can be negatively affected after treatment with methotrexate. Treatment of breastfeeding mothers with methotrexate is not recommended. The retinoids, particularly etretinate (Tegison), have been found to be effective but they have so many untoward effects that they are seldom used. Side effects include lipid abnormalities, calcification of tendons, teratogenicity, and a half-life of more than 120 days. The use of etretinate during breastfeeding should be discouraged. Tazarotene is an effective retinoid for psoriasis and fortunately does not penetrate skin effectively, hence milk levels would likely be minimal. Transcutaneous absorption is less than 1%. Virtually none is detected in the plasma. While it is teratogenic in pregnant women, it is not likely to cause untoward effects in a breastfed infant. But caution is recommended.

Suggested Reading:

1.   Feldman SR, et al. Psoriasis. Med Clin North Am. 1998 Sep;82(5):1135-44, vi.

Review.
2. de Jong EM. The course of psoriasis. Clin Dermatol. 1997 Sep-Oct;15(5):687-92. Review.
3. Stern RS. Psoriasis. Lancet. 1997 Aug 2;350(9074):349-53. Review.
4. Guzzo C. Recent advances in the treatment of psoriasis. Dermatol Clin. 1997 Jan;15(1):59-68. Review.
5. De Tran QH, Guay E, Chartier S, Tousignant J. Tacrolimus in dermatology. J Cutan Med Surg. 2001 Jul-Aug;5(4):329-35. Review.
6. Assmann T, Homey B, Ruzicka T. Topical tacrolimus for the treatment of inflammatory skin diseases. Expert Opin Pharmacother. 2001 Jul;2(7):1167-75.
7. Christophers E. Psoriasis--epidemiology and clinical spectrum. Clin Exp Dermatol. 2001 Jun;26(4):314-20. Review.
8. Skaehill PA. Tacrolimus in dermatologic disorders. Ann Pharmacother. 2001 May;35(5):582-8. Review.

Radiopaque/Radiocontrast Agents

Principles of Therapy:

Radiopaque or radiocontrast agents (except barium) are iodinated compounds used to visualize various organs during X-ray, MRI scans, CAT scans, and other radiological procedures. These compounds are highly iodinated benzoic acid derivatives. Although under usual circumstances, iodine products are moderately contraindicated in nursing mothers (due to ion trapping in milk), these products are unique in that the iodine is covalently bonded to the benzene ring and as such is not metabolized, nor free for transport into milk or the thyroid. According to several manufacturers, less than 0.005% of the iodine is free for transfer into tissues. Further, the bioavailability of most of these compounds is poor to nil, hence they can be used orally as radiopaque agents to visualize the gut. While dozens of these compounds are available, most have not been specifically studied in breastfeeding mothers. Those that have been studied do not appear to penetrate milk effectively.

RADIOPAQUE AGENTS
AAP: Compatible

Trade: Conray, Cholebrine, Telepaque, Oragrafin, Bilivist, Hypaque, Gastrografin, Renovue-Dip, Angiovist, Optiray , etc.

Can/Aus/UK:

Specifics: In one study, the amount of iohexol and metrizoate secreted in breastmilk was less than 0.5% of the maternal dose. According to several manufacturers, less than 0.005% of the iodine is free. These contrast agents are in essence pharmacologically inert, not metabolized, and are rapidly excreted by the kidney (80-90% with 24 hours). They are known to pass unchanged into human milk after IV administration. They are virtually unabsorbed after oral administration(< 0.1% absorption). Most are cleared for pediatric use.

$T\frac{1}{2}$= < 2 hours   Oral= nil   Peak= 1 hour
LRC= L2

IOHEXOL
AAP: Not Reviewed

Trade: Omnipaque
Can/Aus/UK:
Specifics: In a study of 4 women who received 0.755 g/kg (350 mg iodine/mL) of iohexol IV, the mean peak level of iohexol in milk was 35 mg/L at 3 hours post-injection. The average concentration in milk was only 11.4 mg/L over 24 hours. Assuming a daily milk intake of 150 mL/Kg body weight, the amount of iohexol transferred to an infant during the first 24 hours would be 3.7 mg/Kg which corresponds to 0.5 % of the maternal dose.

T½= 2 hours   Oral= Nil   Peak= 3-10 minutes
LRC= L2

METRIZOATE   AAP: Not Reviewed

Trade: Isopaque
Can/Aus/UK:
Specifics: In a study of 4 women who received metrizoate 0.58 g/Kg (350 mg Iodine/mL) IV, the peak level of metrizoate in milk was 14 mg/L at 3 and 6 hours post-injection. The average milk concentration during the first 24 hours was only 11.4 mg/L. During the first 24 hours following injection, it is estimated that a total of 1.7 mg/Kg would be transferred to the infant which is only 0.3% of the maternal dose.
T½= <2 hours   Oral= 60-75%   Peak= Nil
LRC= L2

Clinical Tips:

While there are more than 25 of these radiopaque agents available, most differ only in iodine content. It is well documented that the iodine is not bioavailable but rather is eliminated with the parent compound. These agents as a whole exhibit poor oral bioavailability, hence they would not likely even be absorbed by a breastfeeding infant. Studies of two of the more prominent agents above used for CAT and MRI scans show milk levels are extremely low and the bioavailability low as well. While most manufacturer's suggest a 24 hour waiting period to reinitiate breastfeeding, there is no clear reason for such a prolonged interruption of breastfeeding. A brief interruption of several hours would be more than sufficient although there are no good data to suggest that even this is required.

Radiocontrast agents and their reported milk concentrations*

Drug	Milk (C_{max})	Clinical Significance	Bioavailability
Gadopentetate	3.09 umol/L	Only 0.023% of maternal dose; total dose = 0.013 umol/24h	0.8%
Iohexol	35 mg/L	Mean milk level was only 11.4 mg/L; virtually unabsorbed	<0.1%
Iopanoic Acid	20.8 mg/19-29 h	Only 0.08% of maternal dose; virtually unabsorbed	Nil
Metrizamide	32.9 mg/L	Only 0.02% maternal dose recovered over 44.3 h; poor oral absorption	0.4%
Metrizoate	14 mg/L	Mean milk level 11.4 mg/24h; only 0.3% of maternal dose	Nil

* Adapted from Hale TW, Ilett KF. Drug Therapy and Breastfeeding: From Theory toClinical Practice, First Edition ed. London: Parthenon Publishing; 2002

Suggested Reading:

1. Nielsen ST et.al. Excretion of iohexol and metrizoate in human breastmilk. Acta. Radiol. 28:523-26, 1987.
2. Fitz-John TP, et.al. Intravenous urography during lactation. Br. J. Radiol 55:603-5, 1982.

Radioactive Procedures

Principles of Therapy:

The use of radioactive isotopes for various treatment and diagnostic procedures is quite common. In general, the radioactive substances used in medicine are comprised of nuclides that decay and produce gamma rays, beta particle emissions, alpha particle emissions, and several other less common radioactive emissions. Radioactive nuclides are in general incorporated into chemical mixtures so that they have affinity for various tissue sites. As such, they are chosen for their specific affinity. For instance, Iodine-131 has a high affinity for thyroid, so it is chosen for its biology in the thyroid gland. Technetium-99 nuclides, when incorporated into varius salt forms, have affinity for bony tissue, tissues that are inflammed, and numerous other sites. Thallium-201 salts have a high affinity for myocardial tissues and can be used to diagnose certain myocardial diseases. While most all radioactive nuclides will pass into milk to some degree, many have very brief half-lives and are of minimal risk to the infant if a brief interruption of breastfeeding is used. Others, such as radioactive iodine, are highly risky and must be carefully used, if at all. A comprehensive table of guidelines for radioisotope use in breastfeeding mothers is provided in the Appendix.

X-RAYS

AAP: Not Reviewed

Trade:
Can/Aus/UK:
Specifics: X-Rays pass directly through tissues and are not retained in the body. Hence, women can breastfeed in most instances following radiotherapy with X-Rays.

T½= N/A   Oral=N/A   Peak= N/A
LRC= L1

TECHNETIUM-99M Pertechnetate

AAP: Compatible with temporary cessation.

Trade:
Can/Aus/UK:
Specifics: Technetium-99M pertechnetate is present in human milk. Recommended interruption of breastfeeding is 12 hours for 440 Mbq (12 mCi) or 24 hours for 1100 Mbq (30 mCi) or higher (NRC guidelines).

T½= 6.02 hours   Oral= Complete   Peak= N/A
LRC= L4

IODINE-123

AAP: Compatible with temporary cessation.

Trade: ^{123}Iodine
Can/Aus/UK: ^{123}Iodine
Specifics: ^{123}I has a short half-life of only 13.2 hours and is radiologically ideal for thyroid and other scans. If radioactive iodine compounds are mandatory for various scanning procedures, ^{123}I should be preferred, followed by pumping and discarding milk for 12 hours for a dose of 150 MBq (4 mCi), or 24 hours for 370 MBq(10 mCi). However, the return to breastfeeding following ^{123}I therapy is somewhat dependent on the purity of this product. During manufacture of radioactive ^{123}I, ^{124}I, and ^{125}I are created in small amounts. If using ^{123}I, breastfeeding should be temporarily interrupted (see NRC table in appendices).
T½= 13.2 hours   Oral= Complete   Peak= N/A
LRC= L4

THALLIUM-201

AAP: Compatible with temporary cessation.

Trade: Thallium-201
Can/Aus/UK:
Specifics: In a study of one breastfeeding patient who received 111 MBq (3 mCi) for a brain scan, the amount of Thallium-201 in breastmilk at 4 hours was 326 Bq/mL, and subsequently dropped to 87 Bq/mL after 72 hours. Even without interrupting breastfeeding, the infant would have received less than the NCRP radiation safety guideline dose for infrequent exposure for a 1 year old infant. The NRC recommends interruption of breastfeeding for 2 weeks following a dose of 110 Mbq (3 mCi).
T½= 73.1 hours   Oral= Complete   Peak= N/A
LRC= L4

Clinical Tips:

As with any medication, exposure of the infant to risk is largely dependent on the dose. It is the same with radiation exposure from radionuclides. However, with radioisotopes it is the radiation hazard rather than the chemical hazard that is paramount. With exception of radioactive ^{131}I or ^{125}I, most mothers can continue to breastfeed their infant following a brief interruption with pumping and discarding of the milk. Both radioisotopes of iodine (^{131}I and ^{125}I) pose significant and long-term hazards which include possible ablation of the infant's thyroid, a future increased risk of thyroid carcinoma in the infant, and an elevated theoretical risk of breast cancer (0.32%) in the mother due to the high dose of ^{131}I reposited in lactating breast tissues. Because of these issues, it is the recommendation of the NRC that breastfeeding mothers should discontinue breastfeeding if ^{131}I is required. It is recommendation of these authors that breastfeeding should be discontinued for several weeks 'prior' to therapy to allow involution of the breasts and reduce exposure of the breast tissues to radioactivity. The NRC table provided in the Appendix provides excellent guidelines on the use of radioisotopes and temporary interruption of breastfeeding as a function of dose.

Suggested Reading:

1. Robinson PS, Barker P, Campbell A, et.al. Iodine-131 in breastmilk following therapy for thyroid carcinoma. J. Nuci. Med. 35:1797-1801, 1994.
2. Palmer, KE. Excretion of 125-I in breastmilk following administration of labeled fibrinogen. Br. J. Radiol. 52:672, 1979.
3. Dydek GJ, Blue PW. Human breastmilk excretion of iodine-131 following diagnostic and therapeutic administration to a lactating patient with Graves' disease. J. Nuclear Med. 29(3):407-10, 1988.
4. Robinson PS, Barker P, Campbell A, et.al. Iodine-131 in breastmilk following therapy for thyroid carcinoma. J. Nuci. Med. 35:1797-1801, 1994.
5. Johnston RE, Mukherji SK, et.al. Radiation dose from breastfeeding following administration of Thallium-201. J. Nucl. Med. 12:2079-2082, 1996.
6. Murphy PH, Beasley CW, et.al. Thallium-201 in human milk: Observations and radiological consequences. Health Physics 56(4):539-541, 1989.

Raynaud's Phenomenon

Principles of Therapy:

Raynaud's phenomenon (RP) is characterized by episodic digital arteriospasm resulting in reduced digital blood flow. Most patients are women between the age of 20-45 years with cold-induced or emotion-induced finger pallor that occurs in cold exposure. Upon rewarming, finger color returns to cyanosis, and subsequently to intense redness (reactive hyperemia). Although the fingers are the most commonly involved, the toes, cheeks, and ears may also be affected. Episodes are most common in northern climates during the winter months. The exact etiology is unknown, but supra physiologic vasoconstrictor responses due to hyperreactive alpha-adrenergic receptor activity may predispose to the syndrome. Treatment is largely palliative and is directed toward reducing the conditions that predispose to the symptoms, namely, reducing cold exposure or emotional situations. Preventive measures include warm clothing and gloves and avoidance of the following: tobacco in all forms, ergot alkaloids (ergotamine, bromocriptine), beta-blockers, oral contraceptives, and sympathomimetic medications (stimulants, pseudoephedrine, phenylephrine, phenylpropanolamine, etc). Patients should also avoid vibrating machinery particularly since 40-90% of loggers and 50% of miners who use vibrating equipment experience RP. Pharmacotherapy is not always effective and often the side effects of the medications preclude continued therapy. Raynaud's syndrome may be the first symptom noted in patients with scleroderma.

CAPTOPRIL   AAP: Compatible
    Trade: Capoten
    Can/Aus/UK: Capoten, Apo-Capto, Novo-Captopril, Acenorm, Enzace, Acepril
    Specifics: Milk levels are very low (4.7 µg/L of milk). No adverse effect in 12 infants studied. Avoid in early neonatal periods, infants may be excessively sensitive.
    T1/2= 2.2 hours   Oral= 60-75%   Peak= 1 hr.
    LCR= L3 if used after 30 days
          L4 if used early postpartum

METHYLDOPA   AAP: Compatible
    Trade: Aldomet
    Can/Aus/UK: Aldomet, Apo-Methlydopa, Dopamet, Novo-Medopa, Aldopren, Hydopa, Nudopa
    Specifics: Reported milk levels are quite low in over 9 patients studied. One case of gynecomastia has been reported (personal communication).

T1/2= 105 min.   Oral= 25-50%   Peak= 3-6 hours
LRC= L2

NIFEDIPINE   **AAP**: Compatible
Trade: Adalat, Procardia
Can/Aus/UK: Adalat, Apo-Nifed, Novo-Nifedin, Nu-Nifed, Nifecard, Nyefax, Nefensar XL
Specifics: Milk levels of this calcium channel blocker are quite low. Doses for Raynaud's syndrome vary from 30-60 mg per day in sustained release formulations
T1/2= 1.8-7 hours   Oral= 50%   Peak= 45 min-4 hours
LRC= L2

TERBUTALINE   **AAP**: Compatible
Trade: Bricanyl, Brethine
Can/Aus/UK: Bricanyl
Specifics: Following the oral administration in mothers, milk levels were minimal. No untoward effects were noted in breastfed infants.
T1/2= 14 hours   Oral= 33-50%   Peak= 5-30 min.
LRC= L2

Clinical Tips:

At present the calcium channel blockers appear most effective (60-70%) and include nifedipine, nicardipine and diltiazem. Nifedipine, having the most potent peripheral action, is considered the agent of choice. There are no data available on nicardipine in breastfeeding mothers, but it is probably reasonably safe. Diltiazem may not be suitable for breastfeeding mothers due to higher milk levels. Methyldopa is about 50% effective in Raynaud's and several studies show low milk levels. Although nicotinic acid is marginally effective (< 40%) its use in high doses could be problematic for a breastfed infant (liver damage). Alpha-adrenergic blockers have not been studied in breastfeeding mothers, but due to incredible potency, they are probably too toxic to risk (prazosin, phenoxybenzamine). The ACE inhibitor captopril is marginally effective (30%). There are numerous other medications that are poorly efficacious and have not been studied in breastfeeding mothers. These include: griseofulvin, papaverine, nitrates, guanethidine, reserpine, prostaglandins (PGI2, PGE1), thyroid, dextran, and pentoxifylline.

Suggested Reading:

1.   Cerinic MM, et al. New approaches to Raynaud's phenomenon. Curr Opin Rheumatol. 1997 Nov;9(6):544-56. Review.
2.   Wigley FM, et al. Raynaud's phenomenon. Rheum Dis Clin North Am. 1996 Nov;22(4):765-81. Review.
3.   Belch JJ, et al. Pharmacotherapy of Raynaud's phenomenon. Drugs. 1996 Nov;52(5):682-95. Review.

Rheumatoid Arthritis

Principles of Therapy:

Rheumatoid arthritis (RA) is a chronic systemic inflammatory disease of unknown etiology which is primarily characterized by joint pain.   Spontaneous partial remissions occur in over 75% of patients, with about 10% progressing on to rapid degenerative arthritis. Treatment is highly varied and depends on the source and site of pain, age, and condition of patient (pregnant, breastfeeding), and length and severity of condition. While the salicylates have for ages been the primary tool for treating RA, their high side effect profile has relegated them to lesser status. Treatment of minor rheumatic pain generally begins with the use of acetaminophen, light doses of aspirin, or more likely, the newer NSAIDs.   With increasing severity, intra-articular injections of steroids may be used.   But none of these agents produce remissions in this syndrome.   The disease modifying antirheumatic drugs (DMARD)(e.g. methotrexate, gold salts, azathioprine, etc) can in some cases reduce or retard destruction of the joint, and with many rheumatologists, are being used far earlier than in the past. Timing is critical. Treatment guidelines emphasize that the initiation of DMARD therapy should not be delayed past 3 months for any patient with an established diagnosis who has ongoing joint pain, morning stiffness, active synovitis, and an elevated ESR (SED rate). However, the use of DMARD drugs in breastfeeding mothers is problematic at best, as many of these drugs are not well studied in breastfeeding mothers and are highly toxic. Their use in breastfeeding mothers is not generally advised.

ACETAMINOPHEN

AAP: Compatible

Trade: Tempra, Tylenol, Paracetamol
Can/Aus/UK: Apo-Acetaminophen, Tempra, Tylenol, Paracetamol, Panadol, Dymadon, Calpol
Specifics: Only minimal amounts are secreted in milk.
T½= 2 hours   Oral= >85%   Peak= 0.5-2 hours
LRC= L1

DICLOFENAC

AAP: Not Reviewed

Trade: Cataflam, Voltaren
Can/Aus/UK: Voltaren, Apo-Diclo, Novo-Difenac, Fenac, Voltarol
Specifics: Levels in milk in one study were undetectable.
T½= 1.1 hours   Oral= Complete   Peak=1 hr. (Cataflam)
LRC= L2

FLURBIPROFEN   **AAP**: Not Reviewed

Trade: Ansaid, Froben, Ocufen
Can/Aus/UK: Ansaid, Froben, Ocufen
Specifics: Reported milk levels in two studies are reported to be exceedingly
low.
T½= 3.8-5.7 hours   Oral= Complete   Peak= 1.5 hours
LRC= L2

HYDROXYCHLOROQUINE   **AAP**: Compatible

Trade: Plaquenil
Can/Aus/UK: Plaquenil, Plaqueril
Specifics: Average milk concentration is 1.1 mg/Liter amounting to about 1/3
the clinical dose recommended for infants.
T½= >40 days   Oral= 74%   Peak= 1-2 hours
LRC= L2

IBUPROFEN   **AAP**: Compatible

Trade: Advil, Nuprin, Motrin, Pediaprofen
Can/Aus/UK: Actiprofen, Advil, Amersol, Motrin, ACT-3, Brufen, Nurofen,
Rafen
Specifics: Ibuprofen is an ideal NSAID for breastfeeding mother, due to short
half-life and minimal breastmilk levels.
T½= 1.8-2.5 hours   Oral= 80%   Peak= 1-2 hours
LRC= L1

KETOROLAC   **AAP**: Compatible

Trade: Toradol, Acular
Can/Aus/UK: Acular, Toradol
Specifics: In a study of 10 patients receiving 10 mg PO four times daily
ketorolac was undetectable in 4 milk samples, and exceedingly low in the other
6 patient samples (5.2-7.3 μg/L). While the manufacturer does not approve use
in breastfeeding mothers, the levels in breastmilk are incredibly low, far too
low to induce clinical effects in a breastfeeding infant.   No evidence of
untoward effects in infants has been published.
T½= 2.4-8.6 hours   Oral= >81%   Peak= 0.5 - 1 hr.
LRC= L2

PIROXICAM
AAP: Compatible

Trade: Feldene
Can/Aus/UK:
Specifics: In studies of 5 patients, breastmilk levels were very low (< 78 μg/Liter milk). However, its long half-life (30-86 hours) is not ideal.
T½= 30-86 hours   Oral= Complete   Peak= 3-5 hours
LRC= L2

PREDNISONE
AAP: Compatible

Trade: Deltasone, Meticorten, Orasone
Can/Aus/UK: Apo-Prednisone, Deltasone, Novo-Prednisone, Sone, Panafcort, Decortisyl, Econosone
Specifics: The transfer of prednisone (PO) into milk is reported to be quite low. Doses as high as 120 mg daily do not produce clinically relevant doses via milk (47 μg/day).
T½= 3 hours(elimination)   Oral= 92%   Peak= 1-2 hours
LRC= L2
         L4 for chronic high doses

TRIAMCINOLONE
AAP: Not Reviewed

Trade: Aristocort
Can/Aus/UK: Aristocort, Kenalog
Specifics: Triamcinolone is considered a moderately potent steroid. It is not known if systemically administered triamcinolone would penetrate milk but obviously some will. Studies with prednisone suggest that steroids have great difficulty entering the milk compartment. Doses of prednisone as high as 120 mg/day failed to produce significant milk levels. While long-term high dose therapy may be hazardous to a breastfed infant, brief therapy with triamcinolone even with higher doses would not likely be hazardous to a breastfeeding infant.
T½= 88 minutes   Oral= Complete   Peak= N/A
LRC= L3

Clinical Tips:
Initial treatment of RA has always included the use of salicylates. However, with the high incidence of side effects, they are seldom used today. Acetaminophen, although not anti-inflammatory, may be useful in some patients and could be used safely in breastfeeding mothers. Of the NSAID family, very few have been studied in breastfeeding mothers, and of these, none are popular with RA patients. All patients respond differently to the various NSAIDs. Most patients try several brands prior to finding one that works best for their specific condition. Ibuprofen, while safe for breastfeeding mothers, requires up to four doses daily and has a rather higher

incidence of renal and GI side effects when used chronically. Diclofenac is reportedly better for the GI tract, but has been reported to induce elevated liver enzymes in some patients. However, diclofenac levels in milk are reportedly small to undetectable. Naproxen is transferred into milk at low to moderate levels. However several reports of GI symptoms in breastfed infants suggest that it should be used only briefly and cautiously. Flurbiprofen and ketorolac have been studied in breastfeeding mothers, and their transmission to milk is very low. Unfortunately, we do not have data on many of the newer, more popular NSAIDS. This does not necessarily preclude their use as long as the infant is closely observed for GI symptoms, cramping, and diarrhea. Therapy of a chronic syndrome with daily prednisone is risky, and the incidence of osteoporosis is high. Low to moderate oral doses of prednisone (10mg/day) (short-term) are useful in some patients and is not a contraindication to breastfeeding. Intra-articular injections of triamcinolone are very effective and seldom lead to systemic steroid side effects if they are used less than 3 or 4 injections per joint per year. Due to the minimal plasma levels attained, the amount of triamcinolone transferred into milk is likely small and would not preclude breastfeeding, just be observant of the infant's growth and development. Of the DMARD drugs, hydroxychloroquine (HCQ) and methotrexate are the only medications that have been studied. HCQ may be used in breastfeeding mothers with close observation of the infant as the dose transferred to the infant is less than one-third of the pediatric dose used in malaria regions. While the studies of methotrexate show milk levels are quite low, the reports of methotrexate storage in mucosal cells in the GI tract of infants is concerning, and we hesitate to recommend the use of methotrexate in breastfeeding mothers. The reported concentration of myochrysine(Gold) in milk is low, but due to its incredibly long half-life (up to 26 days), it may not be advisable to expose an infant for long periods to this potentially toxic compound.

Suggested Reading:

1. Schuna AA. Update on treatment of rheumatoid arthritis. J Am Pharm Assoc (Wash). 1998 Nov-Dec;38(6):728-35; quiz 735-7. Review.
2. Gay S. Rheumatoid arthritis. Curr Opin Rheumatol. 1998 May;10(3):185-6. Review.
3. Gremillion RB, et al. Rheumatoid arthritis. Designing and implementing a treatment plan. Postgrad Med. 1998 Feb;103(2):103-6, Review.
4. Aletaha D, Smolen JS. Advances in anti-inflammatory therapy. Acta Med Austriaca. 2002;29(1):1-6. Review.
5. Rahman A, Ahmed S, Underwood M. Disease-modifying drugs in rheumatoid arthritis. Practitioner. 2001 Dec;245(1629):1018-25. Review.

Rosacea

Principles of Therapy:

Rosacea is a chronic inflammatory skin disease primarily affecting the face. This disorder is common in middle-aged and older individuals (30-50 years), and characterized by exaggerated blushing or rosy hue of the cheeks, nose and chin. Although sometimes called adult acne, it is not related. Follicular obstruction and comedones are not present in this disorder. It is instead an inflammatory disorder, characterized by telangiectasis, erythema, inflammatory papules, and pustules appearing in the central areas of the face. Tissue hypertrophy, particularly of the nose (rhinophyma), may result. The cause is unknown but is most common in people with fair complexions. Facial skin is unusually sensitive to skin sensitizers such as harsh soaps, abrasive cleaners, or those containing astringents. While this condition cannot be cured, effective treatments are available. Treatment generally consists of topical metronidazole gel, or oral antibiotics, particularly tetracycline. There are strong indications that depression may play a significant role in the incidence of rosacea. Many dermatologists are now using antidepressants as an adjunctive treatment.

CLINDAMYCIN LOTION/GEL   AAP: Compatible

Trade: Cleocin T
Can/Aus/UK: Dalacin T Topical Solution
Specifics: Systemic absorption is < 0.2%. Milk levels would be nil.
T½= 2.9 hours   Oral= 90%   Peak= 1 hour
LRC= L3

METRONIDAZOLE TOPICAL GEL   AAP: Not Reviewed

Trade: MetroGel Topical
Can/Aus/UK: Metro-Gel, Metrogyl, MetroGel
Specifics: Topical application does not produce systemic absorption.
T½= 8.5 hours   Oral= Complete   Peak= N/A
LRC= L3

CLARITHROMYCIN   AAP: Not Reviewed

Trade: Biaxin
Can/Aus/UK: Biaxin, Klacid
Specifics: Levels in milk are unknown, but most macrolide antibiotics are cleared for use in breastfeeding mothers.   Clarithromycin is preferred over tetracyclines for use in this syndrome in breastfeeding patients.

T½= 5-7 hours   Oral= 50%   Peak= 1.7 hours
LRC= L2

ERYTHROMYCIN

AAP: Compatible

Trade: E-Mycin, Ery-tab, Ery C, Ilosone
Can/Aus/UK: E-Mycin, Ery C, Erythromid, Novo-Rythro, PCE, Ilotyc, EMU-V, Ilosone, EES, Erythrocin, Ceplac, Erycen
Specifics: Reported milk levels are less than 1.5 mg/Liter, generally considered subclinical. Dose for treating Rosacea is 500 mg twice daily.
T½= 1.5-2 hours   Oral= Variable   Peak= 2-4 hours
LRC= L1

TETRACYCLINE

AAP: Compatible

Trade: Achromycin, Sumycin, Terramycin
Can/Aus/UK: Achromycin, Aureomycin, Tetracyn, Mysteclin, Tetrex, Tetrachel
Specifics: Milk levels are low, and oral bioavailability in milk is low. In a study of 5 lactating women receiving 500 mg PO four times daily, the breastmilk concentrations ranged from 0.43 mg/L to 2.58 mg/L. Levels in infants were below the limit of detection. Chronic use over months may not be advisable due to dental staining/altered growth rate.
T½= 6-12 hours   Oral= 75%   Peak= 1.5-4 hours
LRC= L2
    L4 if used chronically

Clinical Tips:

First-line therapy is avoidance of factors that provoke flushing such as heat, sunlight, and ingestion of hot beverages, spicy foods, and alcohol. Topical metronidazole gel 0.75% (MetroGel) or Clindamycin lotion 1% (Cleocin T) are the preferred therapies for rosacea and would be ideal for breastfeeding mothers. Systemic absorption of topical metronidazole or clindamycin is very low to nil. After control, the dose of topical metronidazole or clindamycin can be gently tapered until the next severe recurrence. In one study, topical clindamycin was equally efficacious with oral tetracycline. More severe cases may require oral erythromycin, clarithromycin, or tetracycline. The dose of oral erythromycin varies from 250-500 mg twice daily. Several more recent studies have suggested that oral clarithromycin (250mg twice daily for 1 month, followed by 250 mg daily for one month) is more efficacious than doxycycline. This would be ideal oral therapy for a breastfeeding mother. While the use of tetracycline is not ideal, the initial dose of oral tetracycline is 250 mg QID and may be decreased later to once daily and continued for up to 1 month. However, the 'chronic' use of oral tetracyclines (> 6 weeks) may be problematic in breastfeeding patients and we do not recommend it. It is true that oral tetracycline, when ingested via milk is poorly bioavailable (< 30-40%). While the absolute level of tetracycline in milk is low (< 2.58 mg/Liter) and bioavailability of this would be only 30-40%, taken over a long period of time (months) the amount of tetracycline reaching the infant could be significant. The newer tetracyclines are even more problematic. The bioavailability of the newer tetracyclines (minocycline, doxycycline) is much higher (80%) even in the presence of calcium salts, so that the chronic use of these tetracyclines should be discouraged in breastfeeding mothers. Further, due to chronic hypersensitivity syndrome, minocycline-induced scleral pigmentation, and acute eosinophilic pneumonia now associated with minocycline use, most dermatologists are using doxycycline for chronic acne or rosacea. If needed, the older tetracyclines should probably be used and in the lowest doses possible. Resistant cases may respond to isotretinoin (Accutane), but we do not believe this drug is safe for breastfeeding mothers and infants although there are no data to suggest this. Remember, topical, particularly fluorinated, steroids aggravate rosacea and are contraindicated. One of the most common reasons for the occurrence of rosacea is steroid-induced rosacea. Recently, there is increasing data to suggest that clinical depression may play a major role in the occurrence of rosacea. Many dermatologists have now begun using antidepressants (SSRIs) in these patients with good results.

Suggested Reading:

1. Wilkin JK. Use of topical products for maintaining remission in rosacea [editorial]. Arch Dermatol 1999 Jan;135(1):79-80.
2. Singer MI. Drug therapy of rosacea: a problem-directed approach. J Cutan Med Surg 1998 Jun;2 Suppl 4:S4-20-3.
3. Litt JZ. Rosacea: how to recognize and treat an age-related skin disease. Geriatrics 1997 Nov;52(11):39-40, 42, 45-7.
4. Litt JZ. Steroid-induced rosacea. Am. Fam. Physician 48(1):67-71, 1993.
5. Terresani, C. Pavesi A, et.al. Clarithromycin versus doxycycline in the treatment of rosacea. Int. J. Derm. 36:938-46, 1997.
6. Lindow KB, Warren C. Understanding rosacea. A guide to facilitating care. Am J Nurs 2001; 101(10):44-51.
7. Bamford JT. Rosacea: current thoughts on origin. Semin Cutan Med Surg 2001; 20(3):199-206.
8. Cuevas T. Identifying and treating rosacea. Nurse Pract 2001; 26(6):13-15.

Scabies and Pediculosis

Principles of Therapy:

Scabies is a transmissible ectoparasite infection characterized by superficial burrows, secondary infection, and intense itching. Scabies is caused by the itch mite Sarcoptes scabiei. The female parasite burrows into the stratum corneum and deposits eggs and feces along the burrow. They are transmitted by skin-to-skin contact. Diagnosis is only confirmed by microscopic observation of skin scrapings. Pediculosis is caused by various species of lice. On the head they are called Pediculus humanus capitis and on the body Pediculosis humanus capitis. Lice are transmitted by body contact and by clothing, combs and hats, and occur without regard to social status. Treatment of scabies and lice is primarily by the use of external insecticides.

PERMETHRIN
AAP: Not Reviewed

Trade: Nix, Elimite, A-200, Pyrinex, Pyrinyl
Can/Aus/UK: Nix, Lyclear, Nix, Pyrifoam, Quellada
Specifics: Permethrin absorption through the skin is less than 2% and is rapidly metabolized and excreted. It is very unlikely to enter milk.
T½= N/A   Oral= N/A   Peak= N/A
LRC= L2

IVERMECTIN
AAP: Not Reviewed

Trade: Mectizan
Can/Aus/UK:
Specifics: Amount transferred into milk is low, at least 10 fold less than maternal dose. Dose transferred via milk is 2.75 µg/kg.
T½= 28   Oral= Variable   Peak= 4 hours
LRC= L3

Clinical Tips:

Permethrin is a synthetic pyrethroid structure derived from the ester pyrethrum, a natural insecticide in plants. Permethrin is very effective against body, head lice, and scabies. It is ideal for breastfeeding mothers, because its transcutaneous absorption is minimal and it is very unlikely to ever enter milk. Further, it is very nontoxic. To use for body and head lice, recommend that the hair be washed with detergent, then saturated with permethrin liquid for 10 minutes before rinsing with water. After 14 days, another treatment is often recommended. For scabies, permethrin cream (Elimite) should be applied head to toe for 8-12 hours prior to rinsing off. The manufacturer does not provide recommendations for infants < 2 months of age, but most clinicians would use it. Reapplication may be required after

7 days if mites reappear.   For resistant scabies, ivermectin (200 µg/ Kg PO, one dose) is the most recent recommendation.   Due to significant transcutaneous absorption and the possibility of seizures, lindane solutions are no longer recommended for breastfeeding mothers.   Some of the most common reasons for treatment failure are: 1) other patient contacts have not been treated, 2) bedding and living areas have not been treated and cleaned, and 3) areas under the toenail and fingernails have not been treated effectively.

Suggested Reading:

1. Jansen T, et al. Rosacea: classification and treatment. J R Soc Med. 1997 Mar;90(3):144-50. Review.
2. Webster GF. Acne and rosacea. Med Clin North Am. 1998 Sep;82(5):1145-54, vi. Review.
3. Chalmers DA. Rosacea: recognition and management for the primary care provider. Nurse Pract. 1997 Oct;22(10):18, 23-8, 30. Review.

Schizophrenic Disorders, Psychoses

Principles of Therapy:

The schizophrenic disorders are a group of syndromes manifested by deranged thinking, mood and behavior, and loss of contact with reality. Symptoms and signs vary enormously even within the individual at different times and can vary from complete catatonic stupor to frenzied excitement. Treatment invariably requires the use of strong neuroleptic drugs such as the phenothiazines, thioxanthenes, butyrophenones, and others. Unfortunately, of the medications used in breastfeeding mothers, these families of drugs are the least studied and understood. Because many of them have major and sometimes irreversible side effects, their use in breastfeeding mothers is of significant concern. The medications presented below are rather limited in number, as we have minimal data in the breastfeeding population.

CHLORPROMAZINE
AAP: May be of concern

Trade: Thorazine, Ormazine
Can/Aus/UK: Chlorpromanyl, Largactil, Novo-Chlorpromazine, Chloractil
Specifics: Small amounts are known to be secreted into milk. Following a 1200 mg oral dose, samples were taken at 60, 120, and 180 minutes. Breastmilk concentrations were highest at 120 minutes and were 0.29 mg/L at that time.
T½= 30 hours   Oral= Complete   Peak= 1-2 hours
LRC= L3

CHLORPROTHIXENE
AAP: Not Reviewed

Trade: Taractan
Can/Aus/UK:
Specifics: In one patient taking 200 mg/day, maximum milk concentrations of the parent and metabolite were 19 µg/L and 28.5µg/L respectively. This is approximately 0.1% of the maternal dose.
T½= 8-12 hours   Oral= < 40%   Peak= 4.25 hours
LRC= L3

CLOZAPINE
AAP: May be of concern

Trade: Clozaril
Can/Aus/UK: Clozaril
Specifics: Clozapine is an atypical antipsychotic drug with remarkable efficacy in otherwise refractory patients. Although it suffers from a significant incidence of agranulocytosis (1-2%), its potency and efficacy eventuated its reemergence in the late 1980s for use in selected resistant patients. In a study

of one patient receiving 50 mg/d clozapine at delivery, the maternal and fetal plasma were reported to be 14.1 ng/mL and 27 ng/mL respectively. After 24 hours postpartum, the maternal plasma level was 14.7 ng/mL and maternal milk levels were 63.5 ng/mL. On day 7 postpartum while receiving a dose of 100 mg/d clozapine, the maternal plasma and milk levels were 41.1 ng/mL and 115.6 ng/mL respectively. From this data it is apparent that clozapine concentrates in milk with a milk/plasma ratio of 4.3 at a dose of 50 mg/d and 2.8 at a dose of 100 mg/d. The change from day one to seven suggests that clozapine entry into mature milk is less. From this data, the weight-adjusted relative infant dose would be 1.2% of the maternal dose.

T½= 8-12 hours   Oral= 90%   Peak= 2.5 hours
LRC= L3

HALOPERIDOL

AAP: May be of concern

Trade: Haldol
Can/Aus/UK: Apo-Haloperidol, Haldol, Novo-Peridol, Peridol, Serenace
Specifics: Milk levels are quite low, even after several weeks of therapy.
T½= 12-38 hours   Oral= 60%   Peak= 2-6 hours
LRC= L2

OLANZAPINE

AAP: Not Reviewed

Trade: Zyprexa
Can/Aus/UK: Zyprexa
Specifics: Olanzapine is a typical antipsychotic agent structurally similar to clozapine and may be used for treating schizophrenia. Preliminary unpublished data from Ilett et.al. suggests that the relative infant dose will be approximately 1.05 +/-0.05% of the maternal dose. In a patient receiving 15 mg/d the average milk level (AUC) was 9.3 µg/L and a milk/plasma ratio of 0.35. The highest milk level observed in this patient was 18 µg/L at 6 hours after dose.
T½= 21-54 hours   Oral= 57%   Peak= 5-8 hours
LRC= L3

RISPERIDONE

AAP: May be of concern

Trade: Risperdal
Can/Aus/UK: Risperdal
Specifics: In a study of one patient receiving 6 mg/day of risperidone at steady state, the peak plasma level of approximately 130µg/L occurred 4 hours after an oral dose. Peak milk levels of risperidone and 9-hydroxyrisperidone were approximately 12 µg/L and 40 µg/L respectively. The estimated daily dose of risperidone and metabolite (risperidone equivalents) was 4.3% of the weight-adjusted maternal dose.

T½= 3-20 hours   Oral= 70-94%   Peak= 3-17 hours
LRC= L3

Clinical Tips:

The amount of data on the phenothiazines is very limited although most papers suggest that the clinical dose transferred is low. Information on chlorpromazine suggests that infants can breastfeed without major complications, due to limited transfer into milk. The only reported side effect has been minimal sedation. Although one report has made the suggestion that phenothiazines may be implicated in an increased risk of sleep apnea and SIDS, in these studies the medication (promethazine) was administered directly to infants (PO) rather than via breastmilk. Therefore, unless the dose via milk is high enough to induce sedation, an elevated risk of SIDS is unlikely. Neuro behavioral development appears normal in a number of these infants exposed to long term phenothiazines via breastmilk. As for haloperidol, levels in milk appear quite low, and this drug would be an optimal choice as a rapid neuroleptic agent. New data on risperidone and olanzapine indicate milk levels are quite low for both these agents. Risperidone(Risperidal) and olanzapine(Zyprexa) are becoming more popular as they do not generally induce tardive dyskinesia, extrapyramidal and other symptoms. Hence, they are replacing the older phenothiazines in treatment of psychosis. New data suggest their milk levels are quite low and they did not affect the infants in these preliminary studies. The older clozapine, despite its rather high incidence of agranulocytosis (1-2%), is still commonly used in treatment-refractory patients. Its use in breastfeeding mothers should be viewed very cautiously, and monitoring of the infant for agranulcytosis is probably mandatory.

Suggested Reading:

1. Canuso CM, et al. The evaluation of women with schizophrenia. Psychopharmacol Bull. 1998;34(3):271-7. Review.
2. Smith TE, et al. Standards of care and clinical algorithms for treating schizophrenia. Psychiatr Clin North Am. 1998 Mar;21(1):203-20. Review.
3. Turner T. ABC of mental health. Schizophrenia. BMJ. 1997 Jul 12;315(7100):108-11. Review.
4. Owens MJ and Rish SC. Atypical Antipsychotics. In: Schatzberg AF, Nemeroff CB, editors: Essentials of Clinical Psychopharmacology. Washington DC, 2001. American Psychiatric Publishing, Inc.

Seizure Disorders

Principles of Therapy:

The term epilepsy denotes any disorder characterized by recurrent seizures. A seizure is a transient disturbance of CNS function due to abnormal neuronal discharge across the brain. Approximately 1% of the population has epilepsy with the incidence of epilepsy higher in children and the elderly. Eighty percent of patients with proper doses of anticonvulsants will remain refractory to convulsive seizures. Seizures have innumerable causes, many of which are not yet understood. Specific types of seizures require specific medications, so the selection of medication largely depends on the type of seizure. The medications listed below are used for many seizures ranging from partial, simple partial, complex partial, absence (petit mal), myoclonic, tonic-clonic, etc. Therefore, it is important to understand that the medications herein listed are for all of the various seizures and may not be interchangeable. Most of these medications have been thoroughly studied and used in breastfeeding women for years, with exception of gabapentin and lamotrigine. These newer and significantly less sedating products have yet to be studied.

CARBAMAZEPINE   **AAP**: Compatible

Trade: Tegretol, Epitol
Can/Aus/UK: Apo-Carbamazepine, Mazepine, Tegretol, Teril
Specifics: Monitor thyroid function and recommend CBC occasionally.
T½= 18-54 hours   Oral= 100%   Peak= 4-5 hours
LRC= L2

ETHOSUXIMIDE   AAP: Compatible

Trade: Zarontin
Can/Aus/UK: Zarontin
Specifics: Transfer is minimal. Maximum neonatal plasma levels were less than 2.9 mg/dL.
T½= 31-60 hours   Oral= Complete   Peak= 4 hours
LRC= L4

PHENOBARBITAL   AAP: Give with caution

Trade: Luminal
Can/Aus/UK: Barbilixir, Phenobarbitone, Gardenal
Specifics: Amount transferred is moderate, expect neonatal plasma levels of about 25% of maternal levels or less. In most studies, plasma levels attained in infant were < 2-4 mg/L compared to therapeutic ranges of 20-40 mg/L.

T½= 53-140 hours   Oral= 80% (Adult)   Peak=8-12 hrs
LRC= L3

PHENYTOIN   AAP: Compatible

Trade: Dilantin
Can/Aus/UK: Dilantin, Novo-Phenytoin, Epanutin
Specifics: Amount transferred in milk is minimal. Infant plasma levels are low to undetectable.
T½= 6-24 hours   Oral= 70-100%   Peak= 4-12 hours
LRC= L2

PRIMIDONE   AAP: Give with caution

Trade: Myidone, Mysoline
Can/Aus/UK: Apo-Primidone, Mysoline, Sertan, Misolyne
Specifics: See phenobarbital.
T½= 10-21 hours (primidone)Oral= 90%   Peak= 0.5-5 hours
LRC= L3

VALPROIC ACID   AAP: Compatible

Trade: Depakene, Depakote
Can/Aus/UK: Depakene, Novo-Valproic, Deproic, Epilim, Valpro, Convulex, Epilim
Specifics: Although an anticonvulsant, valproic acid is gaining favor as a first line treatment for mania because it has a broader index of safety than lithium. Monitor liver function.
T½= 14 hours   Oral= Complete   Peak= 1-4 hours
LRC= L2

LAMOTRIGINE   AAP: Not Reviewed

Trade: Lamictal
Can/Aus/UK: Lamictal
Specifics: In a study of a 24 year old female receiving 300 mg/day lamotrigine during pregnancy, maternal serum levels and cord levels of lamotrigine at birth were 3.88 μg/mL in the mother and 3.26 μg/mL in the cord blood.   By day 22, the maternal serum levels were 9.61 μg/mL, the milk concentration was 6.51 mg/L, and the infant's serum level was 2.25 μg/mL. Following a reduction in dose, the prior levels decreased significantly over the next weeks. The milk/plasma ratio at the highest maternal serum level, was 0.562. The estimated dose to infant would be approximately 2-5 mg per day assuming a maternal dose of 200-300 mg per day. The infant developed normally in every way. In another study of a single mother receiving 200

mg/day lamotrigine, milk levels of lamotrigine immediately prior to the next dose (trough) at steady state were 3.48 mg/L (13.6 µM). The authors estimated the daily dose to the infant would be 0.5 mg/kg/day. The manufacturer reports that in a group of 5 women(no dose listed), breastmilk concentrations of lamotrigine ranged from 0.07-5.03 mg/L. Breastmilk levels averaged 40-45% of maternal plasma levels. No ill effects were noted in the infants. In a study by Ohman of 9 breastfeeding women at 3 weeks postpartum, the median milk/plasma ratio was 0.61, and the nursed infants maintained lamotrigine concentrations of approximately 30% of the mother's plasma levels. The authors estimated the dose to the infant at >= 0.2-1 mg/kg/d. No adverse effects were noted in the infants.

T½= 24 hours   Oral= 98%   Peak= 1-4 hours
LRC= L3

GABAPENTIN   AAP: Not Reviewed

Trade: Neurontin
Can/Aus/UK: Neurontin
Specifics: No published data are available on this drug, but its lack of significant sedation may suggest it may be suitable for breastfeeding women. In preliminary results from two patients studied in our own laboratories, milk levels were modest. In one breastfeeding mother who was receiving 1800 mg/d, milk levels were 11.1, 11.1, 11.3, and 11.0 mg/L at 0, 2, 4, and 8 hours, respectively, following a dose of 600 mg. The maternal and infant plasma levels at 2 hours post dose were 16.6 mg/L and less than 0.3 mg/L respectively. In another mother receiving 2400 mg/d milk levels were 4.6, 9.8, 9.0, and 7.2 mg/L at 0, 2, 4, and 8 hours respectively, after a dose of 800 mg. The maternal plasma level at 2 hours post dose was 15.1 mg/L. Using these limited data, the calculated relative infant doses were approximately 6.0% to 3.1% respectively, of the weight-adjusted maternal dose. No adverse events were noted in either of these two infants.

T½= 5-7 hours   Oral= 50-60%   Peak= 1-3 hours
LRC= L3

TOPIRAMATE   AAP: Not Reviewed

Trade: Topamax
Can/Aus/UK: Topamax
Specifics: Topiramate is a new anticonvulsant used in controlling refractory partial seizures. In a group of 2 women receiving topiramate(dose unreported) at three weeks postpartum, the maternal serum levels were 6.3 and 17 umol/L, and milk levels were 7.6 and 15 umol/L respectively. Thus the milk/plasma ratio varied from 0.9 to 1.2. Infant serum levels reported were 1.4 and 1.6 umol/L respectively. Maternal/infant serum ratios were much lower at 0.1 to 0.2. Topiramate has become increasingly popular due to its fewer adverse side

effects. The fact that the plasma levels found in breastfeeding infants were significantly less than in maternal plasma, the risk of using this product in breastfeeding mothers is probably acceptable. Close observation for sedation is advised.

T½= 18-24 hours   Oral= 75%   Peak= 1.5-4 hours

LRC= L3

Clinical Tips:

Phenytoin is an old and efficient anticonvulsant. Present studies show that the amount transferred into milk is rather low and may be too low to be detected in most infants. Published milk levels suggest levels in the range of 0.26 to 1.5 mg per liter of milk. If maternal plasma levels are kept in the 10 mcg/mL range, the amount transferred to the infant should be very low. Carbamazepine is an excellent anticonvulsant, particularly in pediatric patients, due to its limited sedative properties. When used in breastfeeding mothers in doses of 200-800 mg/day, breastmilk levels varied from 1.3 to 3.6 mg per liter of milk. Plasma levels in these infants were subclinical, less than 1 μg/ml. Accumulation in the infant has not been reported. While carbamazepine may induce blood dyscrasia in adults, it has not been reported in children. Phenobarbital has been studied extensively in breastfeeding women. The amount ingested by breastfeeding infants varies from 2 to 4 mg per day. While in an older infant this may not prove problematic, in a newborn it could produce accumulation the first month postpartum. Further, the half-life of phenobarbital in newborns is quite long (100-500 hours) and some accumulation and sedation has been reported. Therefore, when using phenobarbital in breastfeeding mothers early postpartum, the infants' plasma levels should be monitored closely for toxic levels. Primidone is metabolized to phenobarbital and should be used with similar precautions to phenobarbital. Valproic acid transfers poorly into human milk. Reported milk levels are generally less than 0.17 to 0.47 mg per liter of milk. No untoward effects have been reported. Peak Ethosuximide levels in milk are 55 mg per liter with reported peak infant plasma levels of 29 μg/mL after one month, which is subclinical. This data suggested that nursing was safe with normal maternal doses of ethosuximide. As for the newer anticonvulsants such as gabapentin(Neurontin), lamotrigine(Lamictal), felbamate(Felbatol), we have no published data thus far on milk or infant plasma levels in breastfeeding situations. It is not likely that these will penetrate into milk in high levels, but we must wait for published documentation to be certain. Topiramate has recently been briefly studied and its milk levels are low. Plasma levels in exposed infants were 10-20% of the mother's plasma levels, which suggests minimal retention by the infant. Finally, one fortunate feature of anticonvulsant therapy is that we have laboratory tests for most of these compounds. When in doubt, the clinician can always test the plasma level of the infant to accurately measure the plasma level of medication.

Suggested Reading:

1. Delanty N, et al. Medical causes of seizures. Lancet. 1998 ;352(9125):383-90. Review.
2. Roth HL, et al. Seizures. Neurol Clin. 1998 May;16(2):257-84. Review.
3. Marks WJ Jr, et al. Management of seizures and epilepsy. Am Fam Physician. 1998 Apr 1;57(7):1589-600, 1603-4. Review.
4. Morrell MJ. Guidelines for the care of women with epilepsy. Neurology. 1998 Nov;51(5 Suppl 4):S21-7. Review.
5. Zahn CA, et al. Management issues for women with epilepsy: a review of the literature. Neurology. 1998 Oct;51(4):949-56. Review.
6. Wallace SJ, et al. Epilepsy--a guide to medical treatment. 1: Antiepileptic drugs. Hosp Med. 1998 May;59(5):379-87. Review.

Smoking Cessation

Principles of Therapy:

Nicotine replacement therapy is designed to replace the plasma levels of nicotine in a form other than tobacco in order to reduce withdrawal symptoms and aid in withdrawal from the use of tobacco. Presently in the USA, nicotine replacements are in the form of chewable gum and nicotine patches for transcutaneous absorption. Nicotine patches are designed to continuously release nicotine into the cutaneous and subcutaneous layers of the skin which then facilitates systemic absorption. Plasma levels attained are determined by the dose in the patch or gum, but in general produce levels significantly less than that obtained by smoking. The dose administered is then gradually reduced. Recently, the introduction of an older antidepressant, bupropion(Wellbutrin, Zyban) in a new dosage form has become very popular for smoking cessation therapy.

BUPROPION
AAP: Not Reviewed

Trade: Wellbutrin, Zyban
Can/Aus/UK:
Specifics: While this drug has a high mil/plasma ratio, it is not detectable in the infants' plasma. Hence the absolute dose via milk is very low. May lower seizure threshold, so do not use in patients subject to seizures. Also, some reports suggest it may lower milk supply so observe mother closely.
T½= 8-24 hours   Oral= N/A   Peak= 2 hours
LRC= L3

NICOTINE PATCHES
AAP: Not Reviewed

Trade: Habitrol, Nicoderm, Nicotrol, Prostep, Nicotine Patches
Can/Aus/UK: Habitrol, Nicoderm, Nicorette, Prostep, Nicotinell TTS
Specifics: Nicotine plasma levels in patch users is only 1/3 that of smoking 1 pack/day. Never use patches and smoke simultaneously.
T½= 2.0 hours(non-patch)   Oral= 30%   Peak= 2-4 hours
LRC= L3

NICOTINE POLACRILEX (GUM)
AAP: Not Reviewed

Trade: Nicorette, Nicorette DS
Can/Aus/UK: Nicorette
Specifics: With nicotine gum, maternal serum nicotine levels average 30-60% of those found in cigarette smokers. While patches (transdermal systems) produce a sustained and lower nicotine plasma level, nicotine gum may produce large variations in peak levels when the gum is chewed rapidly, fluctuations

similar to smoking itself. Mothers who choose to use nicotine gum and breastfeed should be counseled to refrain from breastfeeding for 2-3 hours after using the gum product.

T½= 2.0 hours   Oral= 30%   Peak= 2-4 hours
LRC= L3

Clinical Tips:

Nicotine patches/gum generally produce plasma levels significantly less than that of smoking one pack of cigarettes daily, so they are in essence preferred over smoking and would offer less risk to a breastfed infant than smoking. It is imperative that the patient be warned to not smoke while using these preparations as plasma nicotine levels could rise dangerously. The use of nicotine patches at night is known to induce nightmares. Removal at bedtime is suggested. A new therapy in the form of an older antidepressant, bupropion, has just been introduced. Current studies suggest an increased rate of smoking cessation with bupropion use (about 15%). Bupropion is a unique case in which the milk/plasma ratio is quite high (2.5 to 8.58), but the absolute amount transferred to milk is quite low as none was detected in the infant. It should not be used in mothers with seizure disorders as bupropion is known to reduce the seizure threshold.

Suggested Reading:

1.   Dale LC, et al. Drug therapy to aid in smoking cessation. Tips on maximizing patients' chances for success. Postgrad Med. 1998 Dec;104(6):75-8, 83-4. Review.
2.   Ritvo PG, et al. A critical review of research related to family physician-assisted smoking cessation interventions. Cancer Prev Control. 1997 Oct;1(4):289-303. Review.
3.   Jorenby DE. New developments in approaches to smoking cessation. Curr Opin Pulm Med. 1998 Mar;4(2):103-6. Review.

Urinary Tract Infection

Principles of Therapy:

Urinary tract infections (UTI) are one of the most common of infections. The term 'Urinary tract infection' encompasses an enormous array of diagnoses including: cystitis, pyelonephritis, bacteruria, infections of catheters, and recurrent infections. Treatment of UTI depends on the delineation of upper or lower tract infection. Lower tract infections are those of the urethra (urethritis) or bladder (cystitis) and are characterized by pyuria, dysuria, frequency or urgency. Upper tract infections, pyelonephritis, my involve both the kidney and bladder. Symptoms include: fever, flank pain, and signs of lower tract infection. Most urinary infections are monomicrobial. The most common bacteria is Escherichia coli, followed by Proteus, Enterobacter, Klebsiella and Pseudomonas species. Infections are generally labeled as an uncomplicated UTI if it occurs in a patient who has no functional or structural anomalies of the kidneys, ureters, bladder, or urethra. Complicated UTIs occur in those patients with structural abnormalities. The incidence of UTI is increased during pregnancy and the post-partum period owing to both the local obstructive effect of the enlarged uterus and to the progesterone effect on ureteral mobility. Urinary stasis is more common and vesicoureteral reflux is more likely to occur. Mild ureteral dilatation and hydronephrosis, especially on the right, may be a normal finding during this time and will usually resort to normal between 2 to 8 weeks post-partum. Additionally, the use of catheterization and birth trauma increase the risk of UTI after delivery. The therapy of an uncomplicated UTI generally requires only 3 days of treatment, while a complicated UTI often requires longer (10 to 14 days) treatment and are often recurrent.

CEFTRIAXONE   **AAP**: Not Reviewed

Trade: Rocephin
Can/Aus/UK: Rocephin
Specifics: Small amounts are transferred into milk (3-4% of maternal serum level). Following a 1 gm IM dose, breastmilk levels were approximately 0.5-0.7 mg/L at between 4-8 hours. The estimated mean milk levels at steady state were 3-4 mg/L. Another source indicates that following a 2 g/d dose and at steady state, approximately 4.4 % of dose penetrates into milk. In this study, the maximum breastmilk concentration was 7.89 mg/L after prolonged therapy (7days). Using this data, the weight-adjusted relative infant dose would only be 0.35% of the maternal dose. Poor oral absorption of ceftriaxone would further limit systemic absorption by the infant.
T½= 7.3 hours   Oral= Poor   Peak= 1 hour
LRC= L2

GENTAMYCIN
AAP: Not Reviewed

Trade: Garamycin
Can/Aus/UK: Alocomicin, Cidomycin, Garamycin, Garatec, Palacos, Septopal
Specifics: The oral absorption of gentamicin (<1%) is generally nil with exception of premature neonates where small amounts may be absorbed. In one study of 10 women given 80 mg three times daily IM for 5 days postpartum, milk levels were measured on day 4. Gentamicin levels in milk were 0.42, 0.48, 0.49, and 0.41 mg/L at 1, 3, 5, and 7 hours respectively. The milk/plasma ratios were 0.11 at 1 hour and 0.44 at 7 hours. Plasma gentamicin levels in neonates were small, were found in only 5 of the 10 neonates, and averaged 0.41 μg/ml. The authors estimate that daily ingestion via breastmilk would be 307 μg for a 3.6 kg neonate (normal neonatal dose = 2.5 mg/kg every 12 hours).

T1/2= 2-3 hours   Oral= < 1%   Peak=
LRC= L2

NITROFURANTOIN
AAP: Not Reviewed

Trade: Furoxone
Can/Aus/UK: Furoxone
Specifics: Following an oral dose, furazolidone is poorly absorbed (< 5%) and is largely inactivated in the gut. Concentrations transferred to milk are unreported, but the total amounts would be exceedingly low due to the low maternal plasma levels attained by this product. Due to poor oral absorption, systemic absorption in a breastfeeding infant would likely be minimal.

T1/2= N/A   Oral= < 5%   Peak= N/A
LRC= L2

OFLOXACIN
AAP: Not Reviewed

Trade: Floxin
Can/Aus/UK: Floxin, Ocuflox, Tarivid
Specifics: In one study in lactating women who received 400 mg oral doses twice daily, drug concentrations in breastmilk averaged 0.05-2.41 mg/L in milk (24 hours and 2 hours post-dose respectively). Milk levels are much lower than ciprofloxacin levels.

T1/2= 5-7 hours   Oral= 98 %   Peak= 0.5-2 hours
LRC= L3

SULFAMETHOXAZOLE
AAP: Not Reviewed

Trade: Gantanol
Can/Aus/UK:
Specifics: Sulfamethoxazole is secreted in breastmilk in small amounts. It

has a longer half-life than other sulfonamides. Use with caution in weakened infants and premature infants or neonates with hyperbilirubinemia.
T1/2= 10.1 hours   Oral= Complete   Peak= 1-4 hours
LRC= L3

TRIMETHOPRIM   AAP: Compatible
Trade: Proloprim, Trimpex
Can/Aus/UK: Proloprim, Alprim, Triprim, Ipral, Monotrim, Tiempe
Specifics: In one study of 50 patients, average milk levels were 2.0 mg/L. Milk/plasma ratio was 1.25. In another group of mothers receiving 160 mg 2-4 times daily, concentrations of 1.2 to 5.5 mg/L were reported in milk.
T1/2= 8-10 hours   Oral= Complete   Peak= 1-4 hours
LRC= L3

TROVAFLOXACIN MESYLATE   AAP: Not Reviewed
Trade: Trovan, Alatrofloxacin
Can/Aus/UK:
Specifics: Reported milk levels are very low and averaged 0.8 mg/Liter of milk. Recent data suggest this product may be hepatotoxic and caution is recommended.
T1/2= 12.2 hours   Oral= 88%   Peak= 1-2 hours
LRC= L4

Clinical Tips:
Initial therapy of uncomplicated acute UTI in breastfeeding mothers is generally trimethoprim/sulfamethoxazole double strength (160/800mg) twice daily for 3 days. Due to the possibility of jaundice and kernicterus, sulfonamides should not be used in premature infants, infants with hyperbilirubinemia or G-6-PD deficiency. They should not be used at term or during the first 30 days postpartum. Nitrofurantoin is another oral therapy useful for uncomplicated lower tract infections. Ofloxacin (300 mg BID) for 3 days is equally effective as the sulfonamides. It is unlikely this brief exposure to this fluoroquinolone would be detrimental to breastfed infants. Due to the emergence of   resistance (30-40% of E.coli), amoxicillin is no longer recommended for UTI. Culture with sensitivity testing is indicated for directing therapy for complicated or recurrent UTI. Treatment of complicated UTI generally requires TMP-SMX or a fluoroquinolone for up to 14 days or longer. This may be slightly more risky for breastfed infants as the emergence of *C. difficile* overgrowth in the infant has been reported, but only in one case.   Caution is urged with longer therapies with the fluoroquinolones. Watch for bloody diarrhea or indications of overgrowth of *C. difficle.* Upper tract infections (pyelonephritis) are predominately caused by *E. Coli.* Outpatient treatment can be given to the non-pregnant patient who does not have evidence of sepsis. TMP-SMX (160/800mg) orally twice daily can be

used for a 14 day course. Sepsis requires hospitalization until afebrile for 24 to 48 hours of antibiotics. Pregnancy may also be an indication for hospitalization. TMP-SMZ, ceftriaxone, gentamycin with ampicillin or a fluoroquinolone may be used though the latter would be less desirable for reasons previously discussed. TMP-SMZ is a less desirable choice near term pregnancy and in the immediate post-partum period due to the competition of sulfonamides with bilirubin and potential for toxicity and kernicterus.

Suggested Reading:

1. Barnett BJ, et al. Urinary tract infection: an overview. Am J Med Sci. 1997 Oct;314(4):245-9. Review.
2. Stapleton A, et al. Prevention of urinary tract infection. Infect Dis Clin North Am. 1997 Sep;11(3):719-33. Review.
3. Hooton TM, et al. Diagnosis and treatment of uncomplicated urinary tract infection. Infect Dis Clin North Am. 1997 Sep;11(3):551-81. Review.
4. Nicolle LE. A practical guide to the management of complicated urinary tract infection. Drugs. 1997 Apr;53(4):583-92. Review.

Venous Thromboembolism

Principles of Therapy:

Venous thromboembolism is a common cause of morbidity and mortality in hospitalized patients. Venous thromboembolism almost invariably starts in the lower limbs and ultimately detaches to cause pulmonary embolism. Consequently, prevention of pulmonary embolism is achieved by preventing deep vein thromboembolism (DVT). Pulmonary embolism is more common in the post-partum period. Patient factors that predispose to thromboembolic disorders include: age over 40, pregnancy, puerperium, recent surgery, orthopedic trauma, immobility, artificial heart valves or atrial fibrillation, and marked obesity. Many hereditary thrombophilia disorders can also now be detected which predispose to thromboembolism. Diagnosis of DVT can be confirmed using a lower extremity doppler study. Diagnosis of PE may require a ventilation – perfusion (V/Q) scan using technetium. Breastfeeding may be restricted for a brief period of time after this study (see section on radioactive procedures). Spiral computed tomography (CT) can also be used in diagnosing PE. Pharmacotherapy of DVT has long included the use of heparin and the vitamin K antagonist (warfarin). However, the newer low molecular weight heparins have significant advantages (longer half-lives, more stable kinetics, fewer bleeds).

HEPARIN   AAP: Not Reviewed
    Trade: Heparin
    Can/Aus/UK:
    Specifics: Heparin is a large molecular weight protein (40,000 daltons) that is not secreted into human milk. Further, it is not orally bioavailable.
    T1/2= 1-2 hours   Oral= None   Peak= 20 min.
    LRC= L1

WARFARIN   AAP: Compatible
    Trade: Coumadin, Panwarfin
    Can/Aus/UK: Coumadin, Warfilone, Marevan
    Specifics: Warfarin is highly protein bound. Milk levels are virtually undetectable. In numerous studies, no effects on breastfeeding infants have been reported.
    T1/2= 1-2.5 days   Oral= Complete   Peak= 0.5-3 days
    LRC= L2

ENOXAPARIN
AAP: Not Reviewed
Trade: Lovenox, Low Molecular Weight Heparin
Can/Aus/UK: Lovenox, Clexane
Specifics: Low molecular fraction (2000-8000 daltons) of heparin. Transfer into human milk is very unlikely due to large molecular weight and no oral bioavailability.
T1/2= 4.5 hours   Oral= None   Peak= 3-5 hour
LRC= L3

DALTEPARIN SODIUM
AAP: Not Reviewed
Trade: Fragmin, Low Molecular Weight Heparin
Can/Aus/UK:
Specifics: In another study of 15 post-caesarian patients following subcutaneous doses of 2500 IU, maternal plasma levels averaged 0.074 to 0.308 IU/mL. Breastmilk levels of dalteparin ranged from < 0.005 to 0.037 IU/mL of milk. Using this data, an infant ingesting 150 mL/kg/day would ingest approximately 5.5 IU/kg/day. Due to the polysaccharide nature of this production, oral absorption is unlikely. The authors suggested that "It appears highly unlikely that puerperal thromboprophylaxis with LMWH has any clinically relevant effect on the nursing infant".
T1/2= 2.3 hours   Oral= None   Peak= 2-4 hours (SC)
LRC= L2

Clinical Tips:
Treatment of DVT primarily rests on the use of anticoagulants such as the warfarin or heparin derivatives. Due to their large molecular weights, heparin and its low molecular weight derivatives, enoxaparin and dalteparin, do not transfer into human milk. Further, they are not orally bioavailable and have not been found to produce side effects in breastfeeding infants. Warfarin derivatives do cross the placenta and are relatively contraindicated during pregnancy. Potential side effects of concern with heparin use include heparin-induced osteoporosis and heparin-induced thrombocytopenia in the mother.

Suggested Reading:
1. Hyers TM. Venous thromboembolism. Am J Respir Crit Care Med. 1999 Jan;159(1):1-14. Review.
2. Clagett GP, et al. Prevention of venous thromboembolism. Chest. 1998 Nov;114(5 Suppl):531S-560S. Review.
3. Goldhaber SZ. Clinical overview of venous thromboembolism. Vasc Med. 1998;3(1):35-40. Review.
4. Thomas DA, et al. Venous thromboembolism. A contemporary diagnostic and therapeutic approach. Postgrad Med. 1997 Oct;102(4):179-81, 185-7, 191-4. Review.

Appendix

Activities of Radiopharmaceuticals That Require Instructions and Records When Administered to Patients Who Are Breast-Feeding an Infant or Child. NRC Regulatory Guide 8.39

Radio-Pharmaceutical	COLUMN 1 Activity Above Which Instructions Are Required		COLUMN 2 Activity Above Which a Record is Required		COLUMN 3 Examples of Recommended Duration of Interruption of Breast-Feeding*
	MBq	mCi	(MBq)	(mCi)	
I-131 NaI	0.01	0.0004	0.07	0.002	Complete cessation (for this infant or child)
I-123 NaI	20	0.5	100	3	
I-123 OIH	100	4	700	20	
I-123 mIBG	70	2	400	10	24 hr for 370 MBq (10mCi) 12 hr for 150 MBq (4 mCi)
I-125 OIH	3	0.08	10	0.4	
I-131 OIH	10	0.30	60	1.5	
Tc-99m DTPA	1,000	30	6,000	150	
Tc-99m MAA	50	1.3	200	6.5	12.6 hr for 150 Mbq (4mCi)
Tc-99m Pertechnetate	100	3	600	15	24 hr for 1,100 Mbq (30mCi) 12 hr for 440 Mbq (12 mCi)

Source: Nuclear Regulatory Commission. For a more complete table see:
Http://neonatal.ama.ttuhsc.edu/lact/radioactive.html

Radio-pharmaceutical	COLUMN 1 Activity Above Which Instructions Are Required		COLUMN 2 Activity Above Which a Record is Required		COLUMN 3 Examples of Recommended Duration of Interruption of Breast-Feeding*
	MBq	mCi	(MBq)	(mCi)	
Tc-99m DISIDA	1,000	30	6,000	150	
Tc-99m Glucoheptonate	1,000	30	6,000	170	
Tc-99m HAM	400	10	2,000	50	
Tc-99m MIBI	1,000	30	6,000	150	
Tc-99m MDP	1,000	30	6,000	150	
Tc-99m PYP	900	25	4,000	120	
Tc-99m Red Blood Cell In Vivo Labeling	400	10	2,000	50	6 hr for 740 Mbq (20 mCi)
Tc-99m Red Blood Cell In Vitro Labeling	1,000	30	6,000	150	
Tc-99m Sulphur Colloid	300	7	1,000	35	6 hr for 440 Mbq (12 mCi)
Tc-99m DTPA Aerosol	1,000	30	6,000	150	
Tc-99m MAG3	1,000	30	6,000	150	

Radio-Pharmaceutical	COLUMN 1 Activity Above Which Instructions Are Required		COLUMN 2 Activity Above Which a Record is Required		COLUMN 3 Examples of Recommended Duration of Interruption of Breast-Feeding*
	MBq	mCi	(MBq)	(mCi)	
Tc-99m White Blood Cells	100	4	600	15	24 hr for 1,100 Mbq (5 mCi) 12 hr for 440 Mbq (2 mCi)
Ga-67 Citrate	1	0.04	7	0.2	1 month for 150 Mbq (4 mCi) 2 weeks for 50 Mbq (1.3 mCi) 1 week for 7 Mbq (0.2 mCi)
Cr-51 EDTA	60	1.6	300	8	
In-111 White Blood Cells	10	0.2	40	1	1 week for 20 Mbq (0.5 mCi)
T1-201 Chloride	40	1	200	5	2 weeks for 110 Mbq (3 mCi)

* The duration of interruption of breast-feeding is selected to reduce the maximum dose to a newborn infant to less than 1 millisievert (0.1 rem), although the regulatory limit is 5 millisieverts (0.5 rem). The actual doses that would be received by most infants would be far below 1 millisievert (0.1 rem). Of course, the physician may use discretion in the recommendation, increasing or decreasing the duration of the interruption.

NOTES: Activities are rounded to one significant figure, except when it was considered appropriate to use two significant figures. Details of the calculations are shown in NUREG-1492, "Regulatory Analysis on Criteria for the Release of Patients Administered Radioactive Material" (Ref.2).

If there is no recommendation in Column 3 of this table, the maximum activity normally administered is below the activities that require instructions on interruption or discontinuation of breast-feeding.

Systematic Equivalencies of Typical Corticosteroids

Glucocorticoid	Approx. Equivalent Dose (mg)	Relative Anti-Inflammatory Potency	Relative Mineralo-corticoid Potency	Half-life	
				Plasma (min)	Biologic (hrs)
Short-Acting					
Cortisone	25	0.8	2	30	8-12
Hydrocortisone	20	1	2	80-118	
Intermediate Acting					
Prednisone	5	4	1	60	18-36
Prednisolone	5	4	1	115-212	
Triamcinolone	4	5	0	200+	
Methyl-prednisolone	4	5	0	78-188	
Long-Acting					
Dexamethasone	0.75	25-30	0	110-210	36-54
Betamethasone	0.6-0.75	25	0	300+	

Potency of Topical Corticosteroids

Steroid	Vehicle

Lowest Potency (may be ineffective for some indications)

0.1%	Betamethasone	cream
0.2%	Betamethasone (Celestone®)	cream
0.04%	Dexamethasone (Hexadrol®)	cream
0.05%	Desonide	cream
0.1%	Dexamethasone (Decadron®, Phosphate, Decaderm®)	cream, gel
1%	Hydrocortisone	cream, ointment, lotion
2.5%	Hydrocortisone	cream, ointment
0.25%	Methylprednisolone acetate (Medrol®)	ointment
1%	Methylprednisolone acetate (Medrol®)	ointment

Low Potency

0.01%	Betamethasone valerate (Valisone®, Reduced Strength)	cream
0.1%	Clocortolone (Cloderm®)	cream
0.01%	Fluocinolone acetonide (Synalar®)	cream, solution
0.025%	Fluorometholone (Oxylone)	cream
0.025%	Flurandrenolide (Cordran®, Cordran®, SP)*	cream, ointment
0.2%	Hydrocortisone valerate (Westcort®)	cream
0.025%	Triamcinolone acetonide (Kenalog®)*	cream

Intermediate Potency

0.025%	Betamethasone benzoate	cream, gel, lotion
0.1%	Betamethasone valerate (Valisone®)*	cream ointment, lotion
0.05%	Desoximetasone (Topicort® LP)	cream
0.025%	Fluocinolone acetonide*	cream, ointment
0.05%	Flurandrenolide (Cordran®, Cordran® SP)*	cream, lotion, ointment
0.05%	Fluticasone propionate (Cutivate®)	cream
0.025%	Halcinonide (Halog®)	cream, ointment
0.1%	Triamcinolone acetonide (Kenalog®)*	cream, ointment

High Potency

0.1%	Amcinonide (Cyclocort®)	cream ointment
0.05%	Betamethasone dipropionate (Diprosone®)	cream ointment, lotion
0.05%	Clobetasol dipropionate	cream ointment
0.25%	Desoximetasone (Topicort®)	cream
0.25%	Diflorasone diacetate (Florone®, Maxiflor®)	cream ointment
0.2%	Fluocinolone (Synalar-HP®)	cream
0.05%	Fluocinonide (Lidex®)*	cream ointment
0.1%	Halcinonide (Halog®)	cream ointment solution
0.05%	Halobetasol propionate (Ultravate®)	cream ointment
0.5%	Triamcinolone acetonide*	cream ointment

From *Medical Letter*, 1982 (Nov 26):104

Therapeutic Drug Levels

Reference (Normal) Values

Drug	Therapeutic Range	
Acetaminophen	10-20	µg/ml
Theophylline	10-20	µg/ml
Carbamazepine	4-10	µg/ml
Ethosuximide	40-100	µg/ml
Phenobarbitol	15-40	µg/ml
Phenytoin		
Neonates	6-14	µg/ml
Children, adults	10-20	µg/ml
Primidone	5-15	µg/ml
Valproic Acid	5-15	µg/ml
Gentamicin		
Peak	5-12	µg/ml
Trough	< 2.0	µg/ml
Vancomycin		
Peak	20-40	µg/ml
Trough	5-10	µg/ml
Digoxin	0.9-2.2	µg/ml
Lithium	0.3-1.3	mmol/L
Salicylates	20-25	mg/dL

From Therapeutic Drug Monitoring Guide, WE Evan, Editor, Abbott Laboratories, 1988.

Typical Radioactive Half-Lives

Radioactive Element	Half-Life
Mo-99	2.75 Days
TI-201	3.05 Days
TI-201	73.1 Hours
Ga-67	3.26 Days
Ga-67	78.3 Hours
I-131	8.02 Days
Xe-133	5.24 Days
In-111	2.80 Days
Cr-51	27.7 Days
I-125	60.1 Days
Sr-89	50.5 Days
Tc-99m	6.02 Hours
I-123	13.2 Hours
Sm-153	47.0 Hours

Managing Hyperbilirubinemia in Healthy Term Newborns: The AAP Practice Standard

Age (hours)	Total Serum Bilirubin (mg/dl)	Recommended Treatment
24 or under		Term infants who are clinically jaundiced at 24 hours of age or under are not considered healthy and need further evaluation
25-48	≥12	Consider phototherapy (based on individual clinical judgement)
	≥15	Phototherapy
	≥20	Exchange transfusion if intensive phototherapy fails*
	≥25	Exchange transfusion and intensive phototherapy
49-72	≥15	Consider phototherapy
	≥18	Phototherapy
	≥25	Exchange transfusion if intensive phototherapy fails
	≥30	Exchange transfusion and intensive phototherapy
Over 72	≥17	Consider phototherapy ·
	≥20	Phototherapy
	≥25	Exchange transfusion if intensive phototherapy fails
	≥30	Exchange transfusion and intensive phototherapy

*Intensive phototherapy should reduce total serum bilirubin by 1-2 mg/dl within 4-6 h. Serum bilirubin should continue to decrease and remain below the threshold level for exchange transfusion. If this does not happen, phototherapy is considered to have failed.
Adapted from American Academy of Pediatrics.

Drug Interactions with Oral Contraceptives

Contraceptives	Anticoagulants Heparin, Warfarin	Oral contraceptives sometimes increase and in some cases decrease clotting factors. Anticoagulant therapy may be altered by addition of contraceptives.
Contraceptives	Barbiturates Griseofulvin Felbamate Carbamazepine Phenytoin Primidone Rifampin	These agents may increase the hepatic cytochrome P450 metabolic enzymes and subsequently reduce levels of estrogens/progestins, thereby reducing efficacy of the oral contraceptives. Pregnancy or symptoms of breakthrough bleeding may occur.
Contraceptives	Antibiotics Griseofulvin Penicillins Tetracycline	Many antibiotics alter gut metabolism of OCs thus reducing their absorption and production of clinical levels. Pregnancy or symptoms of breakthrough bleeding may occur.
Contraceptives	Benzodiazepines Lorazepam Oxazepam Temazepam Alrazolam Diazepam Triazolam	OCs may enhance the metabolism and excretion of lorazepam, temazepam or oxazepam. OCs may also inhibit metabolism of certain benzodiazepines such as: alprazolam, diazepam, triazolam. This may lead to increased half-lives and reduced clearance.
Contraceptives	Beta-Blockers Tricyclics Antidepressants Caffeine Steroids Theophylline	OCs may reduce metabolism and clearance of these agents thus leading to increased plasma levels and side effects.
Contraceptives	Smoking	Smoking significantly increases the risk of major cardiovascular side effects. This is a function of number of cigarettes/day and age.

Guidelines for Glucose Monitoring and Treatment of Hypoglycemia in Term Breastfed Neonates*

Clinical Manifestations of Hypoglycemia

It cannot be emphasized enough that all the clinical signs of hypoglycemia are non-specific, and the physician must assess the general status of the infant by observation and physical examination to rule out disease entities and processes that may need additional laboratory evaluation and treatment.

Some common signs include:
1. Tremors, irritability, jitteriness, exaggerated reflexes
2. High pitched cry
3. Seizures
4. Lethargy, listlessness, limpness, hypotonia
5. Cyanosis, apnea, irregular rapid breathing
6. Hypothermia, temperature instability, vasomotor instability
7. Poor suck and refusal to feed

Management of Documented Hypoglycemia

Asymptomatic Infant
1. Continue breastfeeding (approximately every one to two hours) or feed expressed breast milk or breast milk substitute (approximately 10-15 ml/kg).
2. Recheck blood glucose concentration before subsequent feedings until value is stable in normal range.
3. If neonate is unable to suck, avoid intragastric feeding and begin intravenous therapy. Such an infant is not normal and requires very careful examination and evaluation in addition to more intensive therapy.
4. If enteral feeding is not tolerated, begin intravenous glucose infusion. Such an infant is not normal and requires careful examination and evaluation as well as more intensive treatment.
5. Intravenous therapy: 2cc/kg of 10% glucose by bolus followed by a continuous infusion of 6-8 mg/kg/min of glucose (approximately 100 cc/kg/day). Repeat serum glucose within 30 minutes, and serially thereafter until stable in normal range.

6. If glucose is low despite oral feedings, begin intravenous 10% glucose infusion of 6-8 mg/kg/min (approximately 100 cc/kg/day)
7. Adjust intravenous rate according to blood glucose concentration.
8. Once blood sugar is stabilized in the normal range, resume breastfeeding and slowly reduce intravenous infusion. Check glucose concentrations before feedings until values are stabilized off intravenous fluid.
9. Carefully document signs, physical examination, screening values, laboratory confirmation, treatment and changes in clinical condition.

Symptomatic Infant

1. Initiate intravenous glucose using 2 cc/kg 10% glucose bolus followed by a continuous infusion of 6-8 mg/kg/min glucose (approximately 100 cc/kg/day). Do not rely on oral or intragastric feeding to correct hypoglycemia. Such an infant is not normal and requires careful examination and evaluation.
2. Encourage frequent breastfeeding after relief of symptoms.
3. Adjust intravenous rate by blood glucose concentration.
4. Once blood glucose is stabilized, resume breastfeeding and slowly reduce intravenous infusion. Check glucose concentrations before feedings until values are stabilized off intravenous fluid.
5. Carefully document signs, physical examination, screening values, laboratory confirmation, treatment and changes in clinical condition.

*Adapted from Academy of Breastfeeding Medicine guidelines. Clinical Protocol # 1, with permission.

Index

Index

Ordering Information

Pharmasoft Publishing
21 Tascocita Circle
Amarillo, Texas USA 79124-7301
8:00 AM to 5:00 PM CST

Call **806-376-9900**
Sales **800-378-1317**
FAX **806-376-9901**

Online Web Orders

http://www.iBreastfeeding.com

Single Copies = $ 24.95 USD
Plus shipping

(Texas Residents add 8.25% sales tax)